OVERCOMING
INFERTILITY
Naturally

OVERCOMING
INFERTILITY
Naturally

KAREN
BRADSTREET

Woodland Books

Table of Contents

Note

This book is not intended to offer assistance to couples with physical abnormali-
ties which would render conception impossible, nor is it intended to substitute for competent medical advice. It is, however, intended to offer
education on natural solutions available to couples with unexplained
infertility, hormone imbalances, nutritional deficiencies, psychological
barriers and other impediments which lie in the realm of self-health-care.

The information herein is solely intended for educational purposes.
Neither the author nor the publisher will be liable for use of the information presented in this book.

Like one out of every five or six couples in the United States today, my husband
and I have faced the emotional turmoil of infertility. I've undergone
many of the tests in the doctors' arsenal—blood tests, physical examina-
tions, and even a CAT scan for a possible tumor in my pituitary gland—
and took a medication to balance my hormones that made my symptoms
worse, and which made me so sick I decided the negative effects out-
weighed the possible benefits.

I got weary of the medical community's philosophy I encountered of
attacking the symptoms and not the causes. When I tried to discuss
nutrition, emotions and possible causes for my symptoms with my doctors so I might correct the problem where it started—not just try to cover
it up—doctors clammed up.

So, like many infertile couples, I embarked on a quest to learn all I
could about infertility. I've talked to other infertile couples. I've spent
several years researching infertility and its various causes. My first sources
were medical journals and scientific books, and I devoured everything I
could get my hands on in hopes of discovering the cause of my own
infertility. In addition to researching, I've cried and prayed and soul-
searched and experienced the emotional depths infertile couples experience.

I have friends who overcame fertility problems with herbs and nutritional supplements, so after exploring what the medical world had to
offer my interest in this fascinating aspect of fertility was fueled. I have
focused my research efforts on learning about the relationship between
nutrition, emotions, and reproduction.

Natural alternatives to overcoming infertility offer much promise.
Scientists are discovering vitamins, for example, that are just as effective
as certain drugs in regulating female hormones. You'll find out more as
you read on.

I feel we should know as much as we can about our own bodies and how they function. We are responsible for our own health, yet in many ways we've transferred that responsibility to doctors, psychiatrists, the government and others. Utilizing the information in this book is a good place to start taking back your control. I've yet to find a book that offers you all the information you'll find here.

Couples desiring a child and finding themselves unable to conceive are willing to try just about anything to achieve the desired pregnancy. It is in the hopes that your dream will come true that I share this information with you.

I'm not trying to create false hopes or capitalize on quackery. On the contrary, I've listened to and read story after story of couples who achieved success with the ideas in this book. I've noticed tremendous improvement in my own life upon implementing natural, nutritionally oriented methods of health care. I want to make the information I've gleaned available to as many infertile couples as possible in the hopes that they'll know there are alternatives they may never learn from their doctor.

Life offers no guarantees, and there's no guarantee this information will help you. But it might—and if it does, you'll have cause for celebration!

Introduction

You've been married two, three or (fill in the blank) years and haven't used birth control, but the stork seems to have crossed your name from his delivery list. Or, you've successfully had children already, but can't seem to get pregnant again. Chances are, you're searching your mind for answers as to what step you should take next.

Should you see a medical doctor, and undergo the exhausting battery of infertility tests designed to isolate the problem? Perhaps you've already been through tests, and the final diagnosis was, "We can't find anything wrong." Or maybe you're been told, "Sorry, but you'll never have children." Fortunately, many couples who have been told they'd never have children have gone on to conceive anyway.

The medical field has much to offer infertile couples in the way of solutions. For example, your doctor can prescribe medication designed to stimulate ovulation, balance your hormones, or help create the environment your body needs to conceive. Often, natural alternatives can do the same thing.

If you have a problem like endometriosis, one of the most common causes of infertility, a doctor can surgically remove the growths and perhaps increase your chances of conception. Cleansing and balancing the body nutritionally can often aid in this situation also.

Perhaps you have a structural problem such as blocked fallopian tubes or a tipped uterus. Here too, doctors can often correct the problem and increase your chances of conceiving the child you so deeply desire. Overcoming structural problems is an area where the medical field can be especially useful.

Unfortunately, medical alternatives for the infertile couple aren't always without a dark side. Many fertility drugs cost between $500 to $1000 or more per cycle.* And if your doctor prescribes fertility drugs,

*Note: A complete listing of the side-effects caused by drugs commonly used to treat infertility appears in Appendix D.

are you willing to risk multiple births? One of the records for multiple births—septuplets—is held by a Southern California woman who used a popular fertility drug to conceive. After medical expenses and funeral bills for four of the children, the couple's medical bill reached between $700,000 and $1 million.

Sometimes the drugs doctors give infertile couples can cause more problems than they solve. For example, I was taking a drug called bromocriptine to lower my prolactin hormone which caused me terrible dizziness, leg cramps, stuffy nose and nausea. It also caused me extreme embarrassment. I was taking the drug my first day on the job as a writer for a health food company. Standing in the doorway of my co-worker's office, I asked him if he knew of any natural alternatives to the drug. I started to feel dizzy, and seconds later woke up on the floor of his office. I regained my strength long enough to sit down, and was talking to him when I began to feel dizzy again. I woke up with my head on his desk and the papers I was holding in my hands were scattered all over the floor. That was definitely my most memorable first day on a job. I resolved then and there to find alternatives to drug therapy.

Infertility tests are another procedure to which infertile couples subject themselves. Unfortunately, some tests aren't even accurate. One of the oldest infertility tests, the postcoital test, incorrectly diagnosed half of all infertile couples studied, according to two researchers at the University of Southern California. The test measures whether there is an adequate number of sperm in vaginal mucus several hours after intercourse. The problem with the test, according to the two doctors in the study, is that no one knows what constitutes an adequate number of sperm.[1] Postcoital tests average $50 each.

Fifty dollars is cheap compared to most infertility tests, which can cost exorbitant amounts of money. Some couples spend $30,000, $40,000 and more in their quest to achieve pregnancy. You can spend thousands of dollars on artificial insemination alone—from $4,000 to $8,000 a try—with only a small chance of conceiving.

There's also the emotional roller coaster ride of getting your hopes up and having them dashed, sometimes time and time again. One woman who suffered from secondary infertility—she had one child—ran the gamut of tests. "I felt like they were always holding a carrot in front of me, so I finally gave up," she said. Several women of my acquaintance have shared the same feelings. Of course, if you conceive, the expense and emotional roller coaster ride are probably worth it to you.

But what if doctors can't find anything wrong, or their solutions to your problems never get the desired results? You can explore natural ways to overcome infertility. Understanding the connection between nutrition and reproduction is a must for the infertile couple. The body is designed to heal itself and sustain a high level of health and will usually do so when the laws of health are followed. The information in this book will help you take back control of your body.

Many couples have had success with the ideas presented in this book. There's no guarantee you will—but then again, you might. And if you do, it'll be worth every minute you spent learning about the relationship between nutrition, emotional well-being and fertility.

1 ——————— What is Infertility?

By *medical definition, infertility is the inability to conceive a child after a year of* unprotected sexual intercourse. About 25 percent of all couples attempting pregnancy will conceive the first month. About 80 percent of all couples will conceive within a year provided they have intercourse two to three times per week. It is not unusual for any "fertile" couple to try for eight to ten months before becoming pregnant.

After a year and beyond, about 5 percent more couples will conceive on their own, with no medical intervention. A certain proportion of couples conceive spontaneously even if they've been infertile for years, whether or not they undergo infertility treatment. The reason for "spontaneous conception" remains a mystery. One woman married at 25 and tried in vain to have children until she was 30 years old. Then she suddenly became fertile and went on to have eight children within a 12-year time span.

According to Machelle M. Siebel, associate professor of obstetrics and gynecology at Harvard, in 1980, out of 28 million couples in the United States, 3 million were sterile, 2.8 million were subfertile and 1.2 million required a substantial time period before conception occurred. In other words, 7 million out of every 28 million people at any given time have fertility problems.[2] That amounts to 25 percent of the population!

First-degree infertility is the term used to describe those who have never had children. Second-degree infertility describes those who have had children but find themselves unable to conceive again at any point in their reproductive lives.

Infertility can be traced to the female about 50 percent of the time, to the male about 40 percent of the time, and to a combination or unknown factors about 10 percent of the time. Unfortunately, despite the statistics, most of society still considers infertility to be the woman's problem.

The incidence of infertility has increased somewhat in the past few decades. According to some reports, the average American male sperm count has decreased by 30 percent since 1950. What have we been doing the past 50 or 60 years that would affect the health of our bodies in such a dramatic way? Some of the answers are explored in this book.

One last important point: Infertility is not sterility. Sterility is the inability to have children. Infertility is simply difficulty in conceiving. Being infertile does not mean you're unable to reproduce; it simply means you might have to work a little harder at it.

2 *The Normal Reproductive Process*

The miracle of life is played out day after day, hour after hour without fanfare. Every living thing contains within it the seeds of reproduction, and the cycle of life and death for plants, insects, mammals, birds and fishes goes on all around us, never ceasing, like the ebb and flow of the tide.

Nature weighs the odds heavily in favor of conception. For example, during intercourse millions of sperm are released with each ejaculation to maximize chances of fertilization. Fallopian tubes and ovaries come in pairs so that if a problem exists with one, another can still function. Hormone factors create conditions that facilitate the union of the egg and the sperm. Still, in such a complex system, many things can go wrong. Some of these factors will be discussed in this chapter.

But first, let's look at what must go right. In order for conception to occur, the following factors must be in place:

- The woman must produce an egg from her ovaries
- The fallopian tubes must be open
- Healthy sperm must reach the egg while it is in the fallopian tubes
- The lining of the uterus must be prepared for implantation of the fertilized egg
- The woman must produce the proper hormones to nourish the fertilized egg after it has implanted
- The man must produce healthy sperm

THE FEMALE

Women are born with as many as 2 million eggs in their ovaries. By the time a girl reaches puberty, that number has decreased substantially. When a girl reaches menstruating age, anywhere from age 11 to age 16 or 17, the reproductive process begins with the release of one of these eggs. The ability to create a new life starts when the pituitary gland, located beneath the brain, stimulates the reproductive system with two hormones: follicle stimulating hormone (FSH) and lutenizing hormone (LH).

FSH and LH are chemical messengers from the pituitary to the ovaries, two pecan-sized organs located on either side of the uterus. The ovaries contain a lifetime supply of eggs. Each egg is enclosed in a "wrapper" known as an ovarian follicle.

Each month, under the influence of FSH, somewhere around 20 follicles begin to develop. After the follicles have been developing for about a week, hormone changes make all but one of the follicles stop growing. Occasionally more than one follicle develops and is fertilized, leading to multiple births (twins, triplets, etc.).

The follicle continues to grow until about the 14th day of the menstrual cycle. At this point it breaks out of the ovary and floats free. Surrounded by sticky fluids, it is picked up by hairlike projections called cilia and moved along on its approximately three-day trek to the uterus. It makes this journey through one of the fallopian tubes.

It is only in the fallopian tubes that fertilization can take place. Before ovulation, the hormone estrogen stimulates the secretion of mucus, which makes the sperm's journey through the cervix and toward the fallopian tubes much easier. Pockets in the cervix collect sperm, which can sometimes wait several days for ovulation to occur. During ovulation, the cervical opening softens and dilates to allow the sperm easier passage. Immediately after ovulation the hormone progesterone prepares the uterine lining for a fertilized egg.

If fertilization does not occur, this lining sloughs off about 14 days after ovulation in what is known as menstruation. This cycle is repeated as many as 400 times during a woman's life, only to be interrupted by pregnancy, serious illness or hormone imbalance.

THE MALE

The man's role in reproduction is mainly centered around sperm production. Sperm are constantly being manufactured within the male by the millions—by some estimates, as many as 72 million per day! In order to be fertile a man's sperm must be plentiful, motile, and properly formed.

Sperm develops in the testes, or testicles, which hang outside the body for a good reason: sperm like a cooler climate. They cannot properly develop in temperatures above 95 degrees. The testicles are maintained at a temperature of about 94 degrees—a "tropical" climate, but still cool enough to favor sperm production. The testicles also produce testosterone, the main hormone involved in male sexual function.

Once sperm mature they move out of the testicles into a tiny tube called the epididymis. The epididymis is about 20 feet long, but is packed into a space about an inch and a half long. In the epididymis the sperm develop motility, or the ability to move. They practice whipping their tails with the same motion they'll use to try to reach the egg.

From the epididymis the sperm travel through a tube approximately 16 inches long called the vas deferens, where they may reside for several months. During sexual excitement nerve signals propel sperm from the vas into the urethra, where it picks up substances that help its transport and balance its acidity.

When the man deposits his approximately 200 million sperm—about a teaspoon or thimbleful—into the vagina during sexual climax, the sperm swim through the cervix on their journey to the egg. Around the time of ovulation, the cervical mucus forms into channels that lead through the cervix and into the uterus. Sperm in this medium can more easily swim along the channels into the fallopian tubes.

The journey for a hardy sperm takes about 60 to 90 minutes. However, millions never reach their destination. Only a few hundred ever reach the egg. Some are killed by acid secretions in the vagina. Others take a wrong turn and swim up the wrong fallopian tube, forever losing their chance to make history. Fertilization occurs when one sperm penetrates the lining of the egg, whereupon chemical changes in the egg stop the passage of other sperm. The fertilized egg continues its journey down the fallopian tube and implants in the uterus.

WHAT CAN GO WRONG

The most common causes of infertility in women are:

- failure to ovulate or produce an egg
- blocked fallopian tubes
- glandular imbalances
- failure of the sperm to pass through the cervix and into the uterus
- psychological factors

The most common cause of infertility in men is defective sperm, resulting from:

- hormone imbalances
- inflammation of the testicles due to mumps, gonorrhea, or tuberculosis
- old age
- elevated temperature of the testicles over a long period of time
- the presence of a variocele (varicose vein on the testicle)

Some couples who, because of chemical incompatibility or psychological factors, are unable to conceive together, can conceive with a different partner (of course, I'm not advocating another partner). And, some couples who have already successfully conceived one or more times can have difficulty conceiving at any point in their reproductive lives.

Each of the common causes of infertility is explored in more detail in the next few pages.

Ovulation Problems

Failure to ovulate due to a hormone imbalance is the most common cause of female infertility. By some estimates, as much as 25 percent of female infertility involves ovulatory factors. The most common causes of ovulatory failure are excessive weight loss or weight gain, excessive exercise, and extreme emotional stress—all factors within a female's control.

A common misconception is that the ovaries take turns releasing an egg each month. Although during the course of a year properly functioning ovaries do release about the same number of eggs each, they don't necessarily take turns. Sometimes an egg isn't released at all. Some women may ovulate only once or twice a year, making timing intercourse for conception extremely difficult. Once they reach their mid-30s, women naturally start releasing fewer eggs and their fertility declines. All of these factors may lower any woman's chances of conceiving.

Hormone Imbalances

The two dominant hormones (aside from FSH and LH) in the female reproductive process are estrogen and progesterone. Simplistically speaking, estrogen dominates the first half of the menstrual cycle, and progesterone dominates the second half.

A common cause of infertility, the lack of sufficient progesterone to maintain pregnancy, is known as a luteal phase defect. The standard procedure doctors use to combat this problem is to give a woman supplementary progesterone. It may be more prudent to discover why the body isn't producing enough progesterone and to correct the problem nutritionally rather than using a Band-Aid approach. Such approaches will be discussed later throughout this book.

Another hormone-related cause of female infertility is too much of the hormone prolactin in the blood. The body produces this hormone to prepare the mother-to-be for breastfeeding, but in a non-pregnant woman prolactin can shut down ovulation. Prolactin levels are affected by drugs, stress, exercise, dietary factors and sleep—all factors within a woman's control. Tumors of the pituitary gland and hypothyroidism can also lead to elevated prolactin. Doctors often prescribe the drug bromocriptine (trade name, Parlodel) to suppress prolactin. Vitamin B6 has been demonstrated to be just as effective. Vitamin B6 will be discussed extensively in the section "Vitamins for Fertility."

Several factors can cause hormone imbalance, including long-term or excessive stress, nutritional deficiencies, drugs, and environmental toxins, all of which are discussed extensively throughout this book.

One factor not often discussed in medical circles is the Candida albicans microorganism, the organism which causes vaginal yeast infections and diaper rash. Many nutritional experts and some medical doctors familiar with the Candida organism recognize that it may be a cause of much chronic and unexplained degenerative, immunological and emotional illness. Let's take a closer look at this insidious microorganism.

Candida Albicans

Candida albicans is a naturally occurring, single-celled fungus which lives in the gastrointestinal and genitourinary tracts, as well as on the skin. These fungi are present in everyone, and only become bothersome when they grow out of control. Unchecked Candida can become debilitating, even fatal, according to many researchers.[3]

The first person to popularize the connection between Candida and illness was C. Orion Truss, a medical doctor of Birmingham, Alabama. In the late 1960s Truss noticed that a woman he treated for a vaginal yeast infection no longer suffered from her usual migraine headaches and depression. Dr. Truss reported his experience at a medical conference in 1978. The relationship between yeast and illness received further publicity with the book *The Yeast Connection* written by William G. Crook, M.D.

Candida problems normally begin in the gastrointestinal and urinary tracts. When the Candida become too numerous and secrete their toxins into the bloodstream, allergic reactions can result such as acne, earaches and sensitivity to fumes. If the organism spreads unchecked it can affect the central nervous system and produce symptoms such as irritability, lethargy and depression. Allowed to progress further it can affect the glands and organs, leading to problems such as hypothyroidism and ovarian failure.

Doctors Edward Winger and Phyllis Saifer, both professors at respected California universities, have extensively studied the Candida microorganism. Dr. Winger, a board-certified clinical pathologist and immunopathology specialist, developed a test which demonstrates that human antibodies directed against the human ovary are present in Candida infections, thus contributing to infertility, premenstrual syndrome, and other menstrual irregularities often found in patients with the Candida syndrome.[4] He found that ovarian disorders are experienced by as many as 75 percent of women with chronic Candida infection.

Dr. Winger also discovered that patients with Candida overgrowth often suffer from dysfunction of the endocrine glands. Complications from Candida's attack on the endocrine system may include hormone imbalances, fertility problems (including miscarriage or spontaneous abortions), endometriosis and reduced sex drive.[5] The two most common endocrine effects of Candida are thyroid problems and inflammation of one or both ovaries (ovaritis).

Several doctors have associated infertility with candidiasis, including the pioneer in the field, Dr. Truss. One study showed that many infertile women were able to conceive when treated for Candida.[6] Lawrence D. Dickey, a medical doctor from Fort Collins, Colorado, "repeatedly speaks of clinical ecologists being able to help infertile couples establish a pregnancy just by starting the woman (or both of them) on the antiyeast program."[7]

Unchecked Candida cells secrete at least 79 toxins, some of which can mimic the brain's neurotransmitters and affect thought processes.

They can also wreak havoc with body chemistry and affect the body in other strange ways. For example, in one instance a three-year-old girl was hit in the abdomen and thereafter began to experience abdominal pain. Tests showed that she had an obstruction of her bile duct, so surgeons removed the obstruction. It turned out to be a mass of Candida cells.[8]

Candida can cause or contribute to the following symptoms:

Possible Symptoms of Candida Overgrowth

- Female problems including PMS, endometriosis, ovarian or uterine fibroids, infertility
- Vaginal and/or rectal itching
- Male problems, including prostatitis
- Irritable bowel
- Acne and other skin problems
- Chronic fatigue
- Hormone imbalance, including thyroid disorders
- Allergies
- Feeling "bad all over" and not being able to explain why
- Feeling especially bad on damp days or around moldy places like cellars and basements
- Above-average discomfort in the presence of perfumes, tobacco smoke or toiletries

Candida infection was relatively rare before 1960. With the widespread use of antibiotics and medications, the organism has become a more prevalent problem. It appears Candida depends on the right conditions to gain a stronghold in the body. Reliance on processed foods and a diet high in refined sugar also contribute to Candida overgrowth.

Once it grows out of control Candida is very hard to combat, as many women can attest. (Men can have it too, although women seem to be more vulnerable to it.) It can recur for years, and treatment with antibiotics can lead to further overgrowth by destroying the beneficial bacteria (acidophilus) which normally keep Candida under control.

Candida is best controlled through diet and proper supplementation. A person suffering from Candida should avoid sweets, foods containing yeast or mold, and foods containing heated oils and other free radicals. It is best to avoid processed foods altogether, if possible.

Over-the-counter yeast remedies include Caprystatin, Kaprycidin-A, Candistat, Tanalbit and Cantrol. Caprylic acid, which these remedies contain, is an excellent supplement to use in conquering Candida overgrowth. Other supplements include the herb pau d'arco, which has antifungal properties; garlic—the undeodorized type; and lactobacillus acidophilus, which can be purchased in health food stores.

Dennis Remington, M.D., who specializes in preventive and nutritional medicine and has treated thousands of patients for Candida writes, "We have now seen hundreds and hundreds of women with various hormonal problems including menstrual irregularities, dysmenorrhea, and PMS who have improved dramatically with simple control measures to treat Candida. Our experience certainly reflects that reported in the medical literature."[9]

The organism has difficulty gaining control in a person with a healthy body. Following the guidelines in the previous paragraphs and those offered throughout this book will help you create a healthy environment within your body. A well-nourished body is less likely to suffer from hormone imbalances, whatever their cause.

Possible Causes of Candida Overgrowth

- Antibiotics*
- Birth-control pills
- Cortisone drugs
- Excessive consumption of sweets
- Excessive consumption of refined, nutrient-deficient foods
- Immune system stress
- Emotional stress

*Main cause

Hypothyroid

The thyroid gland, located at the base of the neck, secretes two hormones that regulate growth, metabolism and development. A deficiency in the secretion of these hormones is known as hypothyroid.

This condition deserves a category of its own, as it may be one of the most common but most easily overlooked causes of infertility. Toward the turn of the century, when a connection between thyroid function and reproduction was first discovered, doctors often prescribed thyroid for female problems and met with wonderful success. According to one of the most well-known pioneers in the area of thyroid problems, Dr. Broda Barnes, "It was generally agreed that correction of thyroid deficiency solved [menstrual abnormalities or reproductive problems]—until about 1940."[10]

I spoke with a doctor in Provo, Utah about thyroid-related infertility. He was in his mid-70s and therefore had been around long enough to know about many "old" remedies. He told me that many old remedies still work—among them, thyroid therapy. "I've worked with a lot of infertility cases. Thyroid has probably solved more infertility problems than all other remedies combined," he said. Doctor Emil Novak of Johns Hopkins University several years ago noted that thyroid medication for sterility and miscarriage is often more effective than any other type of treatment.[11] Other noted doctors several decades ago expressed similar opinions.

According to the doctor I spoke with, who had practiced gynecology for several decades, thyroid therapy for infertility and menstrual problems has been almost lost in the flurry of modern medicine. In fact, I had to call several doctors before finding one that even took the connection seriously.

Some doctors aren't even aware there is a connection between thyroid function and female concerns. One woman experiencing secondary infertility told me her doctor said thyroid function had nothing to do with menstruation or fertility, despite overwhelming, documented evidence to the contrary! She had a goiter (a classic symptom of thyroid imbalance) and took thyroid for three months. She noticed a change in her menstrual pattern while taking the preparation, and felt convinced her doctor was wrong but, nevertheless, stopped taking thyroid.

Some doctors are catching on. In his book *Neutraerobics*, Jeffrey Bland, Ph.D., mentions a study of 150 women, aged 24 to 34, who were infertile because they weren't ovulating. Upon testing, many were found to be hypothyroid. When they were treated for hypothyroidism, most showed improved ovulation and some became pregnant. "The investigators conclude that subclinical hypothyroidism may be of greater importance in infertile women with menstrual disorders than is usually thought," Bland concluded.[12]

The reason hypothyroid can lead to infertility, according to Barnes, is because proper amounts of thyroid secretion seem to be necessary for development of the egg and for proper secretion of ovarian hormones. Barnes speculates that if thyroid function is low an egg may be discharged, but it may not be capable of being fertilized or of nesting. Perhaps this is one reason hypothyroid women are susceptible to miscarriage.

Hypothyroid men can also become subfertile. Low thyroid function in men affects sperm production. Studies have shown that when an infertile man is proven to be hypothyroid, treatment for the condition often restores fertility.

Why doesn't thyroid deficiency in infertility cases get more attention? According to Doctor Barnes, a prime reason is because modern thyroid tests often fall short in adequately identifying thyroid function, and these are what most doctors rely on. After many years of practice with thyroid-related disorders, Barnes developed a simple test which proved to be a very reliable indicator of thyroid function. You can do the test yourself at home. All you need is a thermometer.

The Barnes Basal Temperature Test

Shake the thermometer down before you go to bed at night. First thing in the morning, before you get out of bed, put the thermometer snugly in your armpit. Leave it there for exactly 10 minutes while you remain in bed. If the thermometer reads below 97.8 several days in a row, you can suspect thyroid deficiency. (Above 98.2 may indicate hyperthyroid.) Women should use the test from about three days after the onset of menstruation rather than just before menstruation, as body temperature rises before menstruation.

You'll have a better chance of finding an audience for your test results among alternative doctors than conventional doctors, although there may be a few among the conventional ranks familiar with Barnes' work. This is not because the test is unreliable, but rather because conventional MDs are often not familiar with it.

If you have a combination of the following symptoms in addition to a low body temperature, you have good reason to suspect hypothyroid:

Symptoms Most Commonly Experienced in Connection with Hypothyroidism

> Constant, unexplainable fatigue
> Extremely dry skin
> Lethargy
> Puffy face or swelling of face
> Sensitivity to cold more than is normal
> Consistently cold hands and feet
> Weight gain although not overeating
> Loss of hair
> Difficult breathing
> Mood swings/emotional instability
> Painful menstruation
> Breast secretion (galactorrhea)
> Brittle nails
> Adult acne

Although you must have a prescription for thyroid medication, thyroid is a natural preparation, dessicated from animal thyroid (if you purchase Armour brand). Synthetic versions of thyroid hormone exist, but a knowledgeable doctor will encourage you to buy the natural brand because it contains complete thyroid. As one doctor pointed out, "There may be some necessary things in there we haven't identified yet."

If you're a first-generation hypothyroid, a simple supplement of kelp may help you overcome the problem. The thyroid largely depends on iodine, of which kelp is one of the richest known sources. The thyroid also depends on vitamins A, B-2, niacin, B-6, B-12, C and E. In some cases, attention to a nutrient-rich diet, proper exercise and control of stress, without thyroid medicine, may be enough to restore normal thyroid function.

The ideal diet for a person struggling with low thyroid function would be patterned after the following:

Breakfast: Fresh fruit, nuts and seeds.

Lunch: Raw fruits or raw vegetable salad.

Dinner: Complex carbohydrates such as baked potatoes, brown rice, or other served with steamed vegetables or salad. Some experts recommend avoiding whole wheat because it is extremely hypoallergenic for many people.

Chronic Miscarriage

Some infertile couples may actually be conceiving but regularly losing the conception. Many women miscarry without ever knowing they were pregnant. Symptoms of miscarriage include passing large clots of blood during menstruation, cramping more than usual, or a late period with heavy bleeding. It is estimated that 10 percent of all pregnancies result in miscarriage.

Thyroid problems—especially hypothyroid—can lead to habitual miscarriage. Miscarriage can also be caused by a defective egg, defective sperm, hormone imbalance, malnutrition and nutritional deficiencies, immune system problems, drugs, trauma, uterine defects and IUDs.

Antibodies

Several hundred thousand couples have difficulty conceiving because some women produce antibodies to their husband's sperm. Some researchers report that this problem may account for up to 10 percent of infertility cases.[13]

The concept shouldn't be surprising, considering the human body's immune system is equipped to recognize and fight off foreign invaders. Interestingly, the World Health Organization has developed vaccines for population control based on the antibody factor.

Combatting this problem often lies within the couple's own power. See *Chapter 5: A Hodgepodge of Helpful Hints.*

Cervical Mucus Problems

Properly functioning cervical mucus serves as a passageway for sperm and acts as a filter to prevent abnormal sperm from making the trek to the egg. However, in some cases cervical mucus can actually become hostile toward sperm.

Some women produce so much cervical mucus at the time of ovulation that it acts almost like a plug or natural diaphragm against the cervix, preventing the passage of sperm. This problem can sometimes be easily corrected. See *Chapter 5: A Hodgepodge of Helpful Hints.*

Studies have also shown that a woman's emotions can play a large role in whether cervical mucus is friendly or hostile toward sperm. See Chapter 6 for more information on the mind-body relationship.

Sperm Clumping, Low Motility, Abnormal Shapes

Problems with sperm account for a large portion of male infertility. In many cases, bringing the quality of sperm up to par lies within the realm of nutritional helps.

Research into male infertility first picked up steam in the 1970s. Before then, the inability to conceive was usually considered a woman's fault. In many cultures if a woman failed to produce offspring, the husband had the right to cast her away and find another wife who could bear him children.

Fortunately for women times have changed, and the man no longer gets off scott-free in fertility problems. Infertility can be traced to the male as often as to the female.

In order to be considered fertile, a man's sperm must meet the given percentages for motility, number and shapes.

Number: A healthy male ejaculate averages about 60 million sperm, but can be as high as 200 million. Twenty million or less is considered functionally sterile. We'll discuss ways to get the sperm count up and things that tend to bring it down throughout the book.

Motility: Spermagglutination, or sperm that clumps together and is unable to swim well, is responsible for as much as 10 percent of male infertility. It is normal for 5 to 10 percent of sperm to clump together. If more than 20 percent of the sperm clump together, fertilization is considered next to impossible. This is another area where natural solutions can make a big difference.

Shape: Sperm come in all shapes and sizes—short tails, long tails, large heads, small heads. Every man's sperm has its share of rejects—ones with two tails or abnormally large heads, for example. If 60 percent of a man's sperm is normal, a man is considered fertile. Nutrition plays a large role in the development of normal, healthy sperm.

Nutritional Deficiencies

The body's different systems are interrelated in such a way that a problem in one system will affect all the other systems. All of the body's systems need certain nutrients in order to function optimally, so singling out certain vitamins and minerals for a particular system may seem a bit ludicrous. However, there are certain nutrients which have been found to particularly influence the health of the reproductive system.

An overall deficiency in nutrients can eventually negatively affect the reproductive system. For example, the endocrine glands, which secrete and control hormones, depend on a correct supply of nutrients, especially trace minerals. Nutritional deficiencies and harmful chemicals can affect the eggs and sperm even before conception occurs.

Science is just uncovering the many ways certain nutrients can enhance and sometimes restore fertility. Some doctors are willing to admit that there are many areas of infertility which remain relatively unknown, including the nutritional connection. And unfortunately, many doctors are admittedly reluctant to recommend vitamins over drugs and surgery, even when the vitamins are proven more effective or just as effective.

Infections

Pelvic inflammatory disease (PID), a modern epidemic, can damage reproductive organs. This disease is caused by various types of bacteria, such as chlamydia and gonorrhea, which work their way into the uterus and sometimes spread further into the ovaries, often creating inflammation and pain in the reproductive organs. Chlamydia affects 4.5 to 10 million people per year.[14]

As many as one in 10 women who contract pelvic inflammatory disease becomes infertile. According to some reports, chlamydia is responsible for causing sterility in 11,000 women each year. Doctors today can treat PID with antibiotics, except in severe cases, which may require surgery. Severe cases may cause irreversible sterility. If you suspect you may be the victim of a sexually transmitted disease, consult your doctor.

Another bacterial infection, identified as T mycoplasma, invades both male and female genital tracts. Its symptoms are mild so many people aren't aware they have it. A doctor practicing at the New York Hospital, Attila Toth, reported several years ago that a third of all childless couples coming to see him suffered from the infection, which can be overcome with antibiotics. Sixty percent of the couples treated for this infection conceive within three years.[15]

Psychological/Emotional Factors

Do you come down with a cold every time your in-laws are due for a visit? Chances are, that's simple proof your emotions affect your body. When it comes to infertility, the mind-body connection is becoming increasingly scientifically documented. An estimated 5 percent of infertility is caused by psychological or emotional factors. See Chapter 6, which is exclusively devoted to this subject, for more information.

Structural Problems

Structural abnormalities account for a significant number of infertility problems. The most common in women are tubal blockage or infection, fibroids, defective uterus, ovarian cysts, and endometriosis. Men commonly experience varioceles or impotence. Many natural-health enthusiasts contend that often these problems have nutritional or emotional causes and solutions.

For example, some experts believe that feeding artificial hormones to commercial farm animals is leading to a high incidence of early adolescence and reproductive problems in young people. Girls as young as 19 or 20 are experiencing fibrocystic breast disease, endometriosis, and even cancer of the reproductive organs. In Puerto Rico, cases of girls with ovarian cysts and enlarged breasts at the tender ages of four and five have been observed. Dr. Saenz de Rodriguez of Puerto Rico, who worked with many of these children, believed they were becoming contaminated with excess estrogen from hormones fed to beef and poultry.[16]

While attending college in Colorado in 1991, my 21-year-old sister knew several girls her age and younger with fibrocystic breast disease and cancers of the reproductive organs. One young girl found out she needed a hysterectomy, and had to accept the fact that she would never have biological children. Can we accept these increasing incidences of reproductive failure and disease as normal?

Natural health proponents claim cutting out meat which has been tainted with artificial hormones and focusing on a natural-foods diet can help the body overcome these imbalances and heal itself.

Endometriosis

Estimated to be the cause in as many as 30 percent of infertility cases, endometriosis is becoming more prevalent, or at least being discovered more due to advanced surgical techniques. At least 12 million American women suffer from this disease—as much as 10 percent of the population.

Endometriosis is tissue which forms weblike growths and scars in various places within the body, most often the reproductive organs and bowels. These undesirable growths can be found on the ovaries, fallopian tubes, ligaments, bowels and, rarely, even on the lungs and various lymph nodes. Endometrial growths on the ovaries are often called "chocolate cysts" because blood the consistency of chocolate syrup accumulates in them each month and they take on a brown color. They can cause from no pain at all to debilitating pain that renders a woman unable to perform her normal activities for several days per month.

Some experts claim the growths act like normal endometrial tissue (the mucus membrane lining the uterus), swelling and bleeding during ovulation and the menstrual cycle. But unlike the regular menstrual flow, endometrial growths don't leave the body. They remain within the body cavity, often causing internal bleeding, scarring, and inflammation. They can anchor themselves to reproductive organs and cause permanent damage.

No consensus exists as to exactly what causes endometriosis. Some believe hormonal factors such as excess estrogen contribute to the abnormal growths. In a few rare cases endometrios has been found in men with high levels of estrogen. Endometriosis is extremely rare after women pass menopause and estrogen levels drop, giving further credence to the excess estrogen theory.

Others think endometriosis may develop because of a problem with the immune system. They suggest that the lymph or blood system gone haywire may transport endometrial cells throughout the body. This theory would explain why endometrial growths can sometimes be found on the lungs or lymph nodes.

The condition may even be genetic. Women who have a first-degree relative with endometriosis are more likely to have the disease.

The theory of "retrograde menstruation" has been advanced by many experts. This theory purports that somehow in those who suffer from endometriosis, part of the menstrual flow backs up into the abdominal cavity and attaches itself to various surfaces, then responds to hormonal stimulation in much the same way the uterine lining does.

A flaw exists in the theory of retrograde menstruation. Researchers have discovered that virtually all women have retrograde menstruation to some degree, so the answer as to why some women are prone to develop endometriosis while others are not remains unsolved.

Another theory, advanced by some natural-health physicians, is that endometriosis is related to the body's inability to properly absorb calcium. Some believe chronic Candida may play a role in endometriosis.

Although a definitive cause has not been pinpointed, experts do know some factors that seem to contribute to endometriosis. One is delayed childbearing into the late twenties and early thirties. The cessation of menstruation and rise in progesterone that occurs during pregnancy seems to exert a protective influence.

Endometriosis is very uncommon in women who begin having children in their late teens and early twenties. For that reason it is often termed "the career woman's disease." The label is inaccurate, as endometriosis can strike girls in their teens, stay-at-home wives, tall women, short women, thin women and fat women. It is no respecter of persons.

Endometriosis manifests several symptoms. The following are the most common:

Symptoms of Endometriosis

- Menstrual cramping that becomes progressively worse as the years pass
- Pain during intercourse
- Lower abdominal pain
- Passage of large clots and tissue (may be brown in color) during menstruation
- Rectal pain during a bowel movement
- Sharp pain shooting down the inner thigh (indicates endometrial growths on the ovary)
- Irritable bowel, especially before and during menstruation and subsiding after the menstrual cycle
- Sharp pain during ovulation
- Infertility
- Lower back pain
- Nausea
- Heavy menstruation

There are several ways in which endometriosis may impair reproduction. Some are backed by substantial research; others remain unproven. A few of these follow:

Structural Damage

Moderate to severe endometriosis can cause significant damage to the fallopian tubes and ovaries. Such damage can interfere with the ability of the fimbria to pick up discharged eggs. Endometriosis can cause adhesions that completely immobilize the ovaries and lead to inflammation that disrupts normal tissue activity. It may also cause the release of an excess of prostaglandins. All of these disruptions of the delicate reproductive process are of concern to the woman desiring to conceive.

Endocrine Disruption

Endometriosis can also cause disruption in the hormonal system. It may cause elevated prolactin, imbalances in the lutenizing hormone, and luteal phase defects. These theories haven't been completely substantiated, but evidence exists to support them.

Spontaneous Abortion

For some reason, women with endometriosis have a higher risk of first-trimester abortions.

Solving The Problem

Given that endometriosis seems to have a negative effect on fertility, what alternatives exist for the woman who suspects that she has endometriosis?

The standard medical methods of dealing with the disease are drugs and surgery. Drug therapy usually consists of birth-control pills or danazol. In both cases, the treatment may be worse than the disease. Danazol's side-effects include, in decreasing order of frequency, weight gain, bloating, decreased breast size, acne, oily skin, abnormal hair growth, headache, deepening of the voice, hot flushes, and muscle cramps. Many women cannot tolerate the side-effects of danazol and discontinue therapy. Birth control pills aren't much better. They can cause weight gain, nausea, breast tenderness, blood clotting, and permanent sterility, among others things.[17]

Laser surgery is the most common surgical method of removing adhesions, but its effectiveness may be overblown. While browsing through the respected *Journal of Fertility and Sterility* one day, which publishes the most up-to-date information in the field, I was surprised to come across two letters-to-the-editor written by doctors. Both stated that laser removal has not been proven to be effective in managing endometriosis. The letter-writers chastised doctors for making too many unsubstantiated claims in favor of surgery, and for performing too many surgeries. I was surprised that these doctors had the humility to admit there is a lot the medical field doesn't know about endometriosis.

Doctor Eric J. Thomas, professor at the Department of Human Reproduction and Obstetrics of Southampton in England, echoed the sentiments of the two doctors:

> *At present it can only be concluded that no study that has been properly controlled has been able to show that the medical treatment of endometriosis improves future fertility. One has also shown that successful treatment does not improve fertility compared with residual endometriosis or unexplained infertility. . .it is as likely to confer a small detriment and the fact that none of the studies has been able to demonstrate a positive benefit inevitably leads to the conclusion that no causal relationship between endometriosis and infertility has been proved.*[18]

The medical treatment of endometriosis can, at best, only curb symptoms temporily. The disease almost inevitably comes back. If you have endometriosis, by all means consult a medical professional. But natural methods of strengthening the body can also help in managing and perhaps overcoming the disease.

Nutrients that may be helpful in managing endometriosis include the following: vitamin E, iron, black currant oil, vitamin B complex and extra B6, vitamin C with bioflavonoids, calcium and magnesium. Herbs that may be helpful are dong quai, red raspberry leaves and Siberian ginseng. These herbs and nutrients are described in more detail in the chapter *The Wonderful World of Herbs.*

Diet can also play a factor in endometriosis, either for good or ill. Caffeine seems to aggravate the pain. Salt, sugar, animal fats, red meats, fried foods, junk foods and hardened fats should be avoided. The diet should consist largely of raw fruits and vegetables, whole grains, raw nuts and seeds.

If you have endometriosis and want to get pregnant, it seems there is always hope. A friend of mine knows a girl who had severe endometriosis but didn't opt for treatment. She "played the field" with men, so to speak, for several years and never conceived. She felt secure that because of her endometriosis, she'd never get pregnant. After several years of her free-wheeling lifestyle, to her shock she unexpectedly became pregnant. I guess the old adage is true: things happen when you least expect them.

I share this example not to promote a promiscuous lifestyle, but to show that you may try for several years to get pregnant and finally end up with a nice surprise.

Variocele

Structural problems are less common for men, but they do exist. Varicose veins (variocele) in the testes are the most common structural problem for males. Most doctors recommend removal of the variocele, but the problem can be overcome nutritionally, as at least one man attests.

The man and his wife had been trying for years to have a baby. Diagnostic tests found the wife to be fertile. Doctors told the husband he had a low sperm count and a variocele. Varioceles raise the temperature of the scrotum and thereby decrease sperm production. Doctors recommended surgery on the husband as the only hope for this couple, and even then gave him only a 50-50 chance of fathering a child.

Disliking the surgery alternative, the husband decided to search for natural alternatives. He sought out a nutritionist, who recommended zinc, vitamin E, folate, and B12 along with other vitamins and minerals. The husband took over 30 vitamins and minerals faithfully. He began to notice an overall increase in his well-being.

After four months on his new nutritional program, the husband went back to his doctor for a semen analysis. The count was high-normal— 220 million healthy, active sperm anxious to impregnate an egg!

The husband's wife began to show signs of morning sickness. She went to the doctor and came back with the good news. She was pregnant! The couple had a healthy son, and at the time of the writing were expecting their second.

The husband concluded his story, "We can't help but think of the childless couples who believe they have no more than the 50/50 chance surgery offered us. We now know there's an alternative that works. It made our children possible." [19]

Impotence

Another problem experienced occasionally by most men at some time in their reproductive lives is impotence, or the inability to get or maintain an erection sufficient for intercourse. An occasional experience with impotence is certainly frustrating, but no cause for alarm. However, the inability to consumate the sexual act would obviously, if it persisted over a period of time, make impregnation impossible.

More than 10 million American men are chronically impotent. Most of them are over 55, and many of them are diabetic. The incidence increases with age, but impotence is not an inevitable consequence of aging. Up until recently it was believed 90 percent of all impotence cases were psychologically caused. Experts have since realized that disease, medications, nutritional deficiencies and other lifestyle factors can also make it difficult for a man to achieve an erection.

Diabetic men commonly struggle with impotence, but some doctors believe this is actually a self-fulfilling prophecy. A man has diabetes and hears that diabetics struggle with impotence, and suddenly, he experiences impotence. In one study of diabetic men, impotency was traced to three primary causes: psychological factors, medications and other diseases. [20] Diabetic men experiencing impotence should see a urologist, as the problem may involve damage to nerves and arteries.

But what if you're not diabetic and impotence is severely affecting your sex life? Some of the modern solutions are quite zany, although probably appreciated by the men they help. One such solution is the inflatable penile implant. Another is the Male Electronic Genital Stimulator, also known as MEGS. This device is inserted into the rectum before intercourse and can be activated by a remote control device that fits into a piece of jewelry. Men claim the devices work, but you may want to try natural alternatives before going to such drastic measures.

Many factors that contribute to impotence are within a man's control.

Some of these are:

- Excessive consumption of alcohol
- The fear of impotence itself
- Medications, including anti-hypertension drugs, anti-ulcer drugs, lithium, anti-depressants and some tranquilizers
- Anger, stress, fatigue, and depression
- Deficiency of zinc, B-6, and molybdenum
- Lack of attraction to partner
- A high-fat, nutrient-poor diet

Nutritional Helps for Impotence

Zinc

Studies show there is a strong link between zinc and male sexuality. Zinc's benefits are elaborated upon later in this book, so I'll only touch upon the subject lightly here. According to Michael Lesser, M.D., who testified before the Senate Select Committee on Nutrition and Human Needs, the soil of 32 states is zinc-deficient, and commercial fertilizers don't provide zinc.[21] Many alternative doctors feel zinc deficiency is at the root of much impotence.

Low-Fat Diet

Another problem that may increase the incidence of impotence is a high-fat diet. The same dietary factors that lead to hardening of the arteries—one of the major health problems in America today—can also lead to impotence by interfering with blood flow to the male organ. According to John A. McDougall, M.D., the first step to treating impotence is to eliminate fat from the diet. A diet rich in starches, legumes, whole grains, vegetables and fruits provides necessary nutrients but cuts down on fat. With proper attention to diet, improvement may happen within days.[22]

Yohimbine Bark

An herbal extract called yohimbine, isolated from the bark of the African yohimbehe tree, appears to help a large percentage of the men who try it. The bark has long been used in Africa as a treatment for impotence. Modern studies have confirmed its effectiveness. Yohimbine extract helped up to 80 percent of the men who tried it in clinical tests, as reported in the *Journal of Urology*.[23] Many health-food stores carry natural yohimbehe bark. It is also sold by prescription under the names Aphrodyne, Yocon and Yohimex.

Vitamin B6

Pyridoxine, or good 'ol vitamin B6, has helped some men overcome impotence. One doctor discovered that doses of 50 milligrams twice daily conquered impotence in some men who were taking phenelzine.[24]

SUMMARY ON THE NORMAL REPRODUCTIVE PROCESS

Reproduction is a complex process. Nature weighs the odds in favor of conception, but in such a delicate system many things can go wrong. Overuse of drugs, structural problems, hormone imbalances and many other factors can affect a couple's ability to conceive. Fortunately, the remedies to many of these problems lie within a couple's own hands.

Fertility Facts

- Female orgasm plays no role in conception.
- If a woman has a menstrual period, she is not necessarily ovulating. The uterine lining can slough off and mimic menstruation even if a woman does not ovulate.
- Many doctors believe the presence of cramps before the menstrual period is evidence ovulation occured.
- Often women worry that they can't get pregnant because all the sperm runs out after intercourse. Experts assure that this fear is completely unsubstantiated.

3 ——— Nutrition for Fertility

In the Biblical account of man's creation, we learn that the human body was made from the dust of the earth, and in a very literal sense this is true. Our bodies are made up of earthy elements, and in order to function effectively they must have the chemicals they need in their proper amounts.

For example, the bones need calcium, among other things; the blood needs iron; the eyes need vitamin A. We need oxygen to breathe, and water for the proper function of everything in our bodies. With these elements our bodies perform many chemical processes vital to survival—respiration, blood circulation, elimination, and so on. If our bodies lack a certain element, deficiency results and the complex chemical processes keeping us alive can short-circuit, resulting in various health problems and even death.

Science has linked many diseases to vitamin and mineral deficiency. More connections are being made all the time. Here are some of the known connections between vitamin deficiency and disease:[25]

Vitamin A Deficiency
>   Poor night vision
>   Reduced immunity
>   Dry eyes, skin and respiratory tissues

Vitamin B1 Deficiency
>   Beriberi
>   Weight loss, poor appetite, loss of strength and nerve tissue
damage

Vitamin B2 Deficiency
>   Scaly lesions in skin folds
>   Mouth irritation
>   Cracking of skin at the corners of the mouth

Nicotinic Acid Deficiency
  Pellagra

Folic Acid Deficiency
  Anemia

Vitamin B6 Deficiency
  Nerve tissue damage
  Irritability
  Nervousness
  Weakness
  Gastrointestinal problems

Vitamin B12 Deficiency
  Pernicious anemia
  Neuritis

Vitamin C Deficiency
  Scurvy
  Easy bruising

Vitamin D Deficiency
  Rickets

Vitamin E Deficiency
  Possible diseases of red blood cells, heart, muscles and
  nerves

Vitamin K Deficiency
  Hemorrhage from mucus membranes
  Faulty blood coagulation

Vitamin deficiencies aren't the only nutritionally related cause of disease. Other dietary factors such as saturated fat, refined sugar and salt have been linked to degenerative diseases. Many forms of cancer have been linked to Western eating habits. For example, Oriental women, who have a very low incidence of breast cancer when following their native diet high in vegetables and low in saturated fats and meats, become equal in risk with American women when they change to a Western diet. Indeed, the connection between diet and health is impossible to ignore—so impossible that it's meriting cover stories on "mainstream" magazines such as *Time* and *Newsweek*.

What does all this have to do with reproduction? It would be illogical to assume that reproduction is unaffected by nutrition. Like the body's other vital functions, reproduction is in part dependent on proper vitamins, minerals, and other nutrients. For example, the glandular system relies heavily on trace minerals to carry out its metabolic functions. Zinc is only one substance found in high quantities in sperm. Scientists have discovered a strong connection between vitamin B6 and estrogen/progesterone balance in females. How many more connections between nutrition and reproduction remain to be discovered? Chances are, future studies will reveal a connection between fertility and nutrition as least as strong as the connection between cancer and nutrition.

Nature teaches many important lessons in the area of nutrition and fertility. For example, in order for a plant seed to grow, the soil needs to be rich in all the nutrients necessary for the plant's growth. Mineral-deficient soils produce either no crops or below-par crops. By adding essential minerals to "barren" soil, growers can make the soil fertile again.

The same is true for animals. To prove this point, Rollin J. Anderson of Sterling, Utah, reported several cases of infertile animals whose fertility was restored with proper mineral supplementation.

Mr. Anderson purchased a Holstein bull which failed to produce any calves. The bull was about to be sent to the slaughterhouse, but Anderson convinced one of the owners to allow him to put some minerals in the bull's feed. In a short time the bull was siring healthy calves and continued to do so for five years.

In another case a 14-year-old racing mare failed to produce any colts. Anderson suggested that the owner add minerals to her diet. He did, and she went on to produce several colts.

Anderson decided to put his minerals to a final test. He took 16 elderly ewes from a herd that were to be destroyed because they were too old to breed, and then purchased an infertile old ram. Skeptics told him he was crazy—that he would get, at most, six lambs out of the 16 ewes. He mineralized the animals' pasture and gave the ram extra mineral supplementation, then let the ram run with the ewes. He reports that the ewes produced 31 lambs the following spring. Remember, these were animals that were to be discarded because they were infertile.[26]

In another study, a selenium-vitamin E combination fed to cattle and ewes reportedly increased the fertilization rate of those animals.[27]

Will what works for plants and animals work for humans? Granted, we are neither plants nor livestock, but we live by many of the same nutritional laws and are equally dependent upon nutrients from the earth for survival. Fortunately, many nutrition-oriented individuals have realized there may be an enormous connection between nutrition and fertility that partly accounts for the decline in fertility over the past several decades. Unfortunately, an infertile couple will have to find most of the information on nutrition themselves; relatively few doctors are interested in the breakthroughs in nutrition and fertility. Surgery and drugs continue to be the mainstay of health care in America.

Just as certain nutrients are necessary for the body's optimal function, certain chemicals can have a negative effect on reproduction as well. For example, smoking, alcohol, excessive caffeine and several prescription drugs have been found to decrease sperm count. We'll explore these adverse substances in more detail shortly.

The increase in infertility today may also be partly linked to the many chemical additives in our foods and beverages, and our reliance on processed foods. We're inundated with chemicals from the minute we get up in the morning to the time we go to sleep. Though we're one of the most overfed nations in the world, our bodies are starving for nutrients.

Consider the number of food additives and other artificial chemicals you're bombarded with in a single day, and add that up over a period of years. You drink chlorine in your drinking water. The foods you eat are filled with pesticides, dyes, artificial flavorings, refined sugars and preservatives. They're processed so that most of the fiber is removed. You brush your teeth with chemically laden toothpaste, spray your hair with formaldehyde-containing hairspray (the substance with which dead bodies are preserved), and sip soda pops which are full of refined sugar or artificial sweeteners created in a laboratory. If you really think about how many artificial chemicals your body is subject to, you'll be amazed that you're even alive, let alone struggling to have a baby!

In the 1970s Dr. Peter Hill, a researcher with the American Health Foundation in New York, found a strong link between nutrition and fertility. He studied hormone levels in women from the Bantu tribe in Africa before and after they switched from their native diet to the traditional Western diet. Hormone changes while the women were on the Western diet revealed a decrease in fertility, the doctor reported to *Prevention* magazine.[28]

So if a healthy diet is so important, why can people using harsh drugs, alcohol, and living off of hamburgers, colas and candy bars successfully reproduce? We can only speculate. Perhaps some people are more sensitive to nutritional deficiencies or have inherited certain vitamin deficiencies which can affect reproduction. Perhaps negative dietary habits have a cumulative effect that takes years to show up. Perhaps some people are more exposed to adverse substances than others. Whatever the case, it has been proven that nutrition plays a vital role in reproduction and the development of a healthy baby.

Many couples successfully conceive after paying more attention to their diets—which can mean eliminating some substances and consuming more of others. In the words of an old popular song, "Accentuate the positive, eliminate the negative." An optimal diet consists of foods in their natural state as much a possible, focusing on whole grains (brown rice, whole wheat bread, etc.), uncooked fruits, raw vegetables, and nuts.

A couple aiming for a nutrient-rich diet should eliminate white flour and white rice, processed sugar, and other processed food as much as possible.

If you're interested in the naturalist approach, consider kicking off your healthy eating habits with what is referred to in natural health circles as a "cleanse." A cleansing diet focuses on all natural foods or juices and is designed to help the body detoxify itself. One woman told me that she became concerned when she still hadn't conceived after eight months of trying. "I went on a juice cleanse, and the next month I was pregnant," she reported. She drank only fruit juices for one week. While the story is purely anecdotal, this woman was convinced the juice cleanse worked. Some sample cleanses and more information on the philosophy behind them are included in Appendix A.

You may want to supplement your diet with vitamins and minerals appropriate for your needs based on what you learn in this book, but remember, the key to optimal nutrition is to eat a diet as natural and as whole as possible. In addition to eating healthy foods, eliminate substances you know are unhealthy, or at least keep your consumption of them in moderation (alcohol, colas, coffee, tobacco, etc.).

In this section, you'll learn specifically about vitamins and minerals related to enhanced fertility for both men and women. You'll also read about those linked to a decrease in fertility. Like the farmer, you'll learn how to make your own "soil" more fertile.

SUBSTANCES TO ELIMINATE

According to doctors Emil Steinberger and James Lloyd, specialists in the field of reproduction, the effects of dietary toxins many not manifest themselves until later in a person's life. One of those manifestations, the doctors conclude, may be reduced fertility or complete sterility. The doctors point out that toxins used by the mother during pregnancy or even used by youth during their crucial reproductive development years may have long-term negative consequences on reproductive capability.

"It should be noted that the effects of a large number of environmental agents on the development of reproductive organs, particularly in the human, remain unexamined," the doctors said.[29]

RECREATIONAL DRUGS

Tobacco, alcohol, caffeine and illegal drugs such as marijuana and cocaine have all been linked to impaired reproductive ability. Let's examine each of these in more detail.

Tobacco

Cigarette smoke contains hundreds of toxic substances, including nicotine, carbon monoxide, radioactive polonium, and benzopyrene. Cigarettes have a known detrimental effect on fertility. Infertility is reported in 46 percent more smokers than non-smokers.

Male tobacco smokers have more abnormal sperm than the average male. The percentage of abnormal sperm is directly related to the number of cigarettes smoked each day. Sperm density of smokers is reduced an average of 22 percent below that of non-smokers.[30]

Smoking has been shown to raise levels of the lutenizing hormone (LH) and lead to a higher-than-average number of ectopic pregnancies. Women smokers have higher rates of amenorrhea and menstrual abnormalities.

Fertility appears to be reduced in women who smoke 16 or more cigarettes per day. In light smokers (up to 20 cigarettes/day) fertility is 75 percent of that of non-smokers. In heavy smokers (more than 20 cigarettes/day) fertility declines to 57 percent of that of non-smokers.[31]

Caffeine

A study done in North Carolina followed 104 women who had trouble conceiving. Half of them were considered high caffeine consumers, drinking one cup of coffee or its equivalent daily. They were half as likely as women who drank less than one cup of coffee or caffeinated beverages daily to become pregnant. A follow-up study showed that women who used little or no caffeine were four times more likely to become pregnant than those who did.

Another study published in the British medical journal *Lancet* followed 100 women who had recently stopped birth control and planned on becoming pregnant. Women who drank a cup of coffee's worth of caffeine daily were only half as likely to conceive in a given month.[32]

Other researchers discovered an increase in spontaneous abortions, stillbirths and premature births among the offspring of men who drank caffeine, even when their wives didn't.[33] Caffeine appears to act directly on spermatogenesis (the production of sperm).

If caffeine led to infertility in everyone, the earth's population would be sparse—so it appears certain individuals are more susceptible than others. More than 600 mg. per day is suspected to be capable of impairing fertility.

Caffeine Content of Commonly Consumed Beverages

12 oz. Pepsi	38 mg.
12 oz. Mountain Dew	54 mg.
12 oz. CocaCola	45 mg.
12 oz. Dr. Pepper	40 mg.
5 oz. instant coffee	60 mg.

Alcohol

Alcohol can also interfere with conception. A gynecologist in Salt Lake City, Utah, told me about a patient who couldn't conceive for 10 years—until she gave up alcohol; then she conceived almost immediately. Men who drink regularly also have a higher-than-average percentage of defective sperm. One researcher concluded that male chronic drinkers can actually become impotent and sterile.[34]

Some doctors theorize that alcohol decreases fertility because it interferes with the conversion of vitamin A, which is necessary for fertility, to its active form in the testicles.

Hold those nightcaps!

MARIJUANA, COCAINE AND OTHER ILLEGAL DRUGS

Studies suggest that marijuana used during the crucial period of adolescence may lead to decreased fertility later in life. Regular marijuana users—such as men smoking marijuana four times per week for six months—had a decrease in sperm numbers in proportion to the amount of marijuana smoked. Heavy users' sperm count dropped to almost zero.[35]

Just about everyone has seen the sad sight of a baby born addicted to cocaine. Cocaine is a central nervous system stimulant and can have debilitating effects on the endocrine system and other functions of the body. Certainly, a couple trying to conceive should abstain from drugs, both for their own health and for that of their potential child.

PRESCRIPTION DRUGS

Adult children of mothers who took the drug DES, a synthetic hormone widely prescribed during the '40s, '50s and early '60s to prevent miscarriage, are showing a higher than average percentage of reproductive problems. To find out if you might be a "DES baby," ask your mother if she took DES when she was pregnant with you. Unfortunately, DES is still added to animal feed in some instances.

Drugs prescribed for ulcers and ulcerative colitis have been linked to lower sperm count and infertility. Two of the most common are Tagamet and Azulfidine. If you're taking a prescription drug, read the label that came with the drug to see if it warns against negative effects on fertility.

Some antibiotics have been linked to decreased fertility. If you're taking an antibiotic, ask your doctor if it has been reported to have any adverse effects on fertility.

Antidepressant drugs have been found to impair fertility in men. Anticonvulsants have been reported to cause menstrual disorders and ovarian dysfunction. The drug chlorpromazine causes endocrine disorders, such as elevated prolactin, in some humans.

Histamines and serotonins caused testicular damage in test rats, and affected endocrine function in men and women tested. Sperm counts went down by as much as 40 percent in men using these drugs, and women developed elevated prolactin.

Birth-control pills have also caused permanent sterility in some cases. More often, they hamper a woman's ability to conceive for several months after they're discontinued.

Because researchers admit to not knowing the long-term effects of most drugs on reproduction, any drug should be considered a potential risk.

WORKPLACE HAZARDS

Decreased fertility has been found in factory workers who handle lead, pesticides, radiation, anesthetic gas, polystyrene, xylene, some solvents, benzene and mercury. Couples desiring pregnancy should take this into consideration if their workplace falls into one of these categories.

If you work in one of these vocations and want a family, you don't necessarily have to quit your job, although the less you're exposed to questionable chemicals the better. Certain nutrients known as antioxidants, such as vitamin C, have shown promise in protecting the body against dangerous chemicals.

Adelle Davis, a certified nutritionist, conducted extensive research on nutrients many years ago. Her works are timeless, and her findings remain valid today. She writes, "Liver damage caused by various industrial poisons—benzene, nitrobenzene, leaded gasoline, and numerous hydrocarbons—has been corrected by diets high in protein and vitamin C."[36] Because the liver is a main organ of detoxification, such findings have an implication for an infertile couple exposed to toxic chemicals.

Men who spend most of their time sitting—truck drivers, office workers, and so on—also tend to have a lower sperm count. This is probably because the testicles remain too close to the body, and the increased heat impairs sperm production.

ENVIRONMENTAL HAZARDS

The pesticides DDT and DCBs have been found to lower fertility in men. So has excessive exposure to lead, plutonium, and dioxyn. Radiation (including X-rays) can cause infertility and even sterility in both men and women. Of all the organs in the body, the reproductive organs are most sensitive to radiation.

A flame retardant used on mattresses, pillows and auto seat covers was reported to possibly lead to a decrease in male fertility in the late '70s and early '80s. The chemical, known as Fyrol FR2, was found in the seminal fluid of one-fourth of the male college students tested at Florida State University in 1980. The chemical is a proven mutagen which can cause genetic damage and birth defects.[37]

Heavy Metals

Many heavy metals have demonstrated negative effects on fertility. Some of these are:[38]

Arsenic: Causes infertility, and is a suspected mutagen and known carcinogen.

Boron: Literature in the former Soviet Union reports infertility, poor sperm development and reduced libido in men exposed to boron.

Cadmium: Although reproductive effects in humans have not been confirmed, in laboratory animals cadmium causes sterility. Case studies suggest a connection between the inhalation of cadmium dust, prostate cancer, and decreased sperm production.

Lead: Men exposed to lead occupationally showed disturbances in the sperm production process, and pregnant women exposed to lead have a higher incidence of stillbirths, spontaneous abortions and low-birth-weight babies.

Manganese: Used as a gasoline additive and in the chemical and steel industries. Men exposed to manganese occupationally demonstrate decreased sex drive and impotence. However, trace amounts of manganese appear to be necessary to reproductive function.

Mercury: Men exposed to inorganic mercury demonstrate loss of sex drive and disturbance in sperm production. Women exposed to mercury report menstrual disorders.

Food Additives

Some food additives are perfectly natural, such as beta carotene, which is added to margarine and other foods for color. However, myriads of additives are not natural and are not fully tested, yet pages of new food additives are approved by the FDA monthly. Although food additives must by law be tested for safety, many tests are incomplete. For example, the body may be able to handle one food additive in minute quantities and therefore the additive is accepted as safe—but what happens when a person consumes additives in almost everything he eats, year after year? What about additives which are safe alone but have a negative reaction in the body when combined with other additives?

Aspartame, for example, most commonly known as NutraSweet™, was tested for a short period of time in the amounts it was believed people would generally consume and pronounced safe, despite the objections of many researchers that it may cause depression, endocrine imbalances, seizures and blindness. People consumed much more NutraSweet than the "experts" anticipated, and hundreds of complaints have been filed against this "safe" substance—some claiming it has caused seizures, blindness, depression, mood swings, and paranoia.

Some substances originally recognized as safe, such as certain food dyes, have later been found to be carcinogenic. Some are actually proven carcinogens in animals, such as saccharin. Of course, the body can probably safely handle one additive here and there, but what happens when everything you eat contains additives and other chemicals?

Some additives have demonstrated negative effects on the reproductive system in test animals. A list of these follows.[39]

BHA: This additive is found in baked goods, baking mixes, beverages, breakfast cereals, candies, chewing gum, gelatins, ice cream, potato chips, shortening and vegetables. It is used to prevent fats and oils from becoming rancid. Tests show that it may cause enzyme changes in the body that adversely affect reproduction.

BHT: Has basically the same effects as BHA, and is used in the same products.

Nitrates and Nitrites: These controversial additives have received a great deal of negative publicity as carcinogens, but they are still used to inhibit botulism-causing organisms and improve the color and flavor of foods. They are mostly used in processed meats such as bacon, hotdogs, lunch meats, sausage, and ham. Some nitrites and nitrates have an adverse effect on fertility, reduce prenatal growth and increase the number of prenatal deaths.

Oxystearin: Found in salad oils; is used to blend and clarify. It may cause testicular cancer.

MSG: A flavor enhancer used in almost all processed and Chinese food; causes many reproductive dysfunctions in test animals. It causes female animals to conceive less frequently and give birth to smaller litters. MSG has also been found to affect neonatal hormones. Because MSG is so widely used in processed foods, it pays to start reading labels if you're having difficulty conceiving.

Growth Hormones

Many animals raised commercially are given hormones (including DES) to make them grow faster. Although the FDA claims these hormones are safe, groups such as the Center for Science in the Public Interest have raised concern about the potential for abusing the use of hormones in cattle.

DES was banned as a carcinogen in the United States and Italy several years ago. However, in the early 1980s calves in Italy were injected with black-marketed DES. The veal was used for baby food and some claimed that babies who ate the baby food grew breasts and girls began to menstruate.

If questions of safety exist, why are artificial hormones used at all? For one thing, they make animals consume less grain and reach market weight sooner. Animals treated with hormones gain more muscle tissue than untreated animals, leading to leaner beef. All of these things amount to about $650 million per year in savings for the beef industry. But pocketbooks aside, if a cow ain't broke, why fix her?

Most hormones and antibiotics given to cattle also find their way into the milk supply. One controversial additive, BGH (bovine growth hormone) has received a great deal of negative publicity. Some dairy farmers have pushed for the use of this hormone in their cattle to make them produce more milk, despite potential harm to human health.

One writer in discussing artificial hormones defies all logic: "...the way cattle today receive hormones is far safer. Instead of injecting these substances into muscle tissue that may be eaten, feedlot operators implant time-release hormone pellets behind animals' ears, which are not used for human food."[40] If the hormones administered only remained behind the animals' ears, what good would they be? Obviously, they must affect the animal's whole body.

Fortunately, certified untreated beef and other untreated animals are available on the market. Consumer awareness is creating a greater demand for untreated animals, and manufacturers are responding. For example, Foster Farms, the poultry manufacturers, base a whole advertisement on the fact that they don't treat their chickens with artificial hormones.

If, after reading this section, you feel like life in the 20th century may be hazardous to your fertility, take heart! Many nutritional factors have been found to protect and heal the body against modern threats. Those discussed in this section show great promise. (For a complete listing of the negative effects of chemicals on reproduction, see "Reproductive Effects of Chemical Agents," Susan D. Schrag and Robert L. Dixon, Reproductive Toxicology, edited by R. L. Dixon, Raven Press, New York, 1985, 301-317)

VITAMINS AND MINERALS FOR FERTILITY

Vitamin B6

Vitamin B6 has been many an infertile woman's best friend. Many female reproductive processes seem to be linked to this vitamin. Deficiencies may cause premenstrual syndrome, hormone imbalance, premenstrual acne, and depression. If you are infertile and suffer from extreme PMS, it may be a sign your body is low on B6. Birth control pills almost completely eliminate this vitamin from the body.

Mounds of research have piled up on the relationship between this vitamin and female fertility. For example, two gynecologists studied 14 women aged 23 to 31 who had unexplained infertility. They all had premenstrual tension. They had been unable to become pregnant anywhere from 18 months to seven years. Doctors gave them from 100 to 800 mg. of B6 daily. Eleven of the 14 became pregnant within six months. One more became pregnant in the seventh, and another in the 11th. One woman dropped out of the study after adopting a child, and another dropped out after a divorce.

Progesterone concentrations increased in five of the seven women whose hormone levels were measured, which Dr. Hargrove, one of the doctors involved, felt may have explained the return of fertility.[41]

B6 and Estrogen/Progesterone Balance

A proper balance between the hormones estrogen and progesterone is essential for pregnancy to occur. Vitamin B6 can play a key role in balancing these two hormones.

When estrogen builds up in the system, the ovary responds by cutting down its production of progesterone, which can lead to chronic abortion and luteal phase defects. Although administering progesterone is the standard medical treatment, a wiser solution might be to discover why the body is not manufacturing enough on its own. Some doctors have begun to recommend vitamin B6 therapy for appropriate hormone-related gynecological problems. Vitamin B6 is often effective in balancing estrogen and progesterone—and it's natural. [42]

A report from New York Medical College pointed out that vitamin B6 corrects estrogen-caused biochemical abnormalities. This is one of the reasons it is often recommended for women with PMS. Excess estrogen can cause the mood fluctuations to which premenstrual women are so subject.

B6 and Elevated Prolactin

Elevated serum prolactin—too much of the hormone prolactin in the blood—is to blame for a significant number of infertility problems. Prolactin is the hormone which prepares the mother-to-be for breastfeeding. Too much of this hormone can prevent a woman from becoming pregnant by interfering with ovulation. Elevated prolactin can also lead to a condition called galactorrhea, or lactation by a non pregnant woman, and cessation of menstruation (amenorrhea).

Doctors often prescribe a drug called bromocriptine to alleviate this condition, but it is not without its side-effects, which include dizziness and fainting, nausea, nightmares, visual disturbances, stuffy nose and leg cramps. Vitamin B6 has been found to be as effective as bromocriptine in lowering prolactin. Perhaps this explains why infertile women on B6 therapy have a high pregnancy rate.

Doctor Jonathan Wright, a nutritionally oriented medical doctor who has used B6 therapy to help hundreds of patients, claimed, "A review of the biochemistry of the bromocriptine drugs shows that pyridoxine (B6) can do all the same jobs they do, and once again with fewer potential side-effects."[43]

Scientists at Harvard treated three women suffering from galactor-rhea-amenorrhea syndrome with supplements of 200 to 600 mg. of vitamin B6 daily. Within three months all three women returned to normal menstruation. When the B6 was stopped, symptoms returned.[44]

Generally, doctors put women with galactorrhea on anywhere from 100 to 800 milligrams of B6 daily. Because too much of one vitamin can cause an imbalance with others, a B-complex supplement should be taken when using extra B6.

Food Sources of B6

Chicken, fish, kidney, liver, pork, eggs, unmilled rice, soy beans, oats, whole wheat products, peanuts, walnuts.

Note: Galactorrhea-amenorrhea can also be caused by hypothyroid. Check with a competent physician if you have this problem and see the section on hyperthyroidism.

Vitamin E

Of all the vitamins, vitamin E is probably the one most mentioned in fertility discussions. Is there any scientific evidence to back the claim that vitamin E enhances fertility? The answer is yes.

Studies have shown that vitamin E can improve sperm's impregnating ability. In several studies, men unable to produce normal sperm were given 150 to 300 IU of vitamin E daily for eight to 40 weeks. Many developed normal sperm and impregnated their wives.[45]

Many nutritional doctors claim vitamin E helps prevent miscarriage by developing a more healthy uterine wall and increasing the health of the placenta. Vitamin E is plentiful in a diet of whole grains, seeds and nuts. When refined, flour, rice and other grains lose most of their vitamin E. White flour loses 92 percent of this vitamin. Almonds, another rich source of vitamin E in their raw state, lose 80 percent of the vitamin in roasting.[46]

In one experiment involving several hundred women who had miscarried two, three or more times, 97 percent delivered healthy babies when undergoing vitamin E therapy.[47] Such tests lead many nutritionists to claim that vitamin E has definitely been proven effective in helping female infertility. Said Carlton Fredericks, Ph.D., "We shouldn't confuse virility with fertility, which is known to be helped by vitamin E."

Wheat germ, which is very rich in vitamin E, has often been recommended for infertile couples as a dietary addition. Dr. Christopher, a well-known nutritionist and Master Herbalist, claimed to help many infertile couples with a diet rich in wheat germ.

Dr. Christopher developed a special diet for couples with problems conceiving. He first recommended that a couple stop eating processed foods and start on a diet with plenty of raw food, with fruits and vegetable juices. Second, he recommended drinking around a gallon of pure water daily. Third, he recommended keeping the bowels in good working order with a good herbal bowel formula. Next, he recommended taking a teaspoon of false unicorn root twice daily. Finally, he recommended a teaspoon of wheat germ oil (rich in vitamin E) three times each day.

"While in my early practice nearly forty years ago," wrote Dr. Christopher, "I would promise a couple that if they would follow this routine they would either conceive or have a baby within a year. Many have accomplished this." One of Dr. Christopher's couples had been married 14 years and had no children. In just a little over a year after following his recommendations, the couple had a baby.[48]

Food Sources of Vitamin E

Wheat germ, whole grains and uncooked nuts.

Zinc

Several studies have shown that zinc plays a key role in the development of healthy sperm. Sperm cells have a greater zinc concentration than any other cell in the body, and a large concentration at that. Zinc affects female fertility as well, especially when taken in combination with B6.

Ali Abbasi, an endocrinologist in Virginia, participated in studies which showed that even a marginal zinc deficiency can cause sperm counts to drop below the point of technical sterility. Abbasi and his colleagues fed a group of men a zinc-deficient diet. Their sperm counts dropped substantially. Upon the addition of supplemental zinc to the men's diets, their sperm count came back to normal.[49]

Low sperm motility has also been shown to improve with added dietary zinc. A urologist named Joel Marmar, from Cherry Hill, New Jersey, claimed to boost sperm motility by as much as 33 percent by giving men with low semen zinc levels supplemental zinc sulfate.

Oysters, long held to be a male aphrodisiac, happen to be very rich in zinc. So are pumpkin and sunflower seeds. So husbands, down those oysters. Maybe there's something to those old wive's tales after all!

Food Sources of Zinc

Seafood, meat and organ meats, nuts and seeds, dairy products, whole grains, brewer's yeast.

Vitamin C

Studies have shown that men with sperm clumping, when given 500 mg. of vitamin C every 12 hours for one month, experienced a drop in these problems from 67 percent clumping to 11 percent. Twenty percent or more is considered infertile.[50]

In a study by Earl B. Dawson, Ph.D. at the University of Texas Medical Branch, Galveston, vitamin C reversed the infertility of 15 men in the petrochemical industry. Within four days of taking the supplemental vitamin C, all of the men showed significant improvements in all the three areas that matter so much: motility, viability and number. The men took one gram (1,000 mg.) of vitamin C daily.[51]

Because spermagglutination is responsible for as much as 10 percent of male infertility, the vitamin C connection is exciting news. Vitamin C supplements are cheap, natural and show a great deal of promise.

Furthering the evidence for vitamin C's beneficial effects on sperm production, researchers at UC Berkeley found that low levels of vitamin C can damage DNA in sperm, resulting in a higher incidence of birth defects, genetic diseases and childhood cancers. When researchers switched men from a high-vitamin-C diet to a vitamin-C-deficient diet, sperm showed increased levels of DNA damage. Upon resupplementing the diet with vitamin C, DNA damage declined. The study was reported in *Men's Fitness*, July 1992.

Is what is true for the goose true for the gander? In this case, yes. Vitamin C also seems to play a role in ovarian function and egg development. A Japanese gynecologist, Masao Igarashi, experimented with vitamin C both by itself and combined with clomiphene, a traditional infertility drug. In two out of five women who failed to ovulate, vitamin C alone prompted ovulation.

Vitamin C with clomiphene corrected ovulation problems in five out of five cases, and worked better than clomiphene alone in many other infertility cases.

Dr. Igarashi reported one case in which a sterile woman who did not respond to drug treatment responded to 400 mg. daily of vitamin C. The vitamin treatment induced ovulation, she conceived, and delivered a normal baby.[52]

As an antioxidant, vitamin C is also under scientific scrutiny for its power to protect the body against many toxic substances. Since we're all exposed to toxins daily which can obviously affect the reproductive process, supplementation is a good idea, especially for men and women who work with harmful substances.

Food Sources of Vitamin C

Asparagus, blackberries, broccoli, cantaloupe, cauliflower, Chinese cabbage, grapefruit, grapefruit juice, kale, kiwi fruit, kohlrabi, mangoes, mustard greens, oranges, orange juice, peppers, raspberries, red cabbage, strawberries, tangerines, tomatoes, tomato juice.

Bioflavonoids

Bioflavonoids are vitaminlike substances found in the white part of fruit rinds and in broccoli, parsley, potatoes, cabbage and green peppers. These nutrients play a role in the formation of healthy blood vessels.

The development of healthy blood vessels is important as the uterus prepares for implantation. If the lining is weak and unhealthy, spontaneous abortion may occur. Bioflavonoids seem to play a role in developing a healthy uterine lining.

In the 1950s researchers at Cornell University studied 100 pregnant women with histories of spontaneous abortion. The women took large doses of bioflavonoids with vitamin C throughout their pregnancies. Ninety-one carried their babies to full term.[53]

Other studies have since been carried out, with similar results. A group of French doctors, headed by Dr. T. Muller, used a bioflavonoid called flavone on a group of women with female problems. They found that flavone compounds were "effective substitutes for hormone therapy in most cases of functional uterine bleeding." Out of 20 women who were treated for irregular menstrual flow not caused by physical damage to reproductive organs, 18 had results rated from good to excellent. Most saw improvement within three menstrual cycles.[54]

Bioflavonoids have been shown to improve the tone of veins and increase the resistance of capillary walls. This is why they seem to help strengthen the uterus after implantation of an egg. Bioflavonoids offer promise in helping to nutritionally strengthen the body against miscarriage.

Food Sources of Bioflavonoids

Broccoli, cabbage, green peppers, parsley, citrus fruit rinds.

B Complex Vitamins

The B complex vitamins are often referred to as the stress vitamins, as they play a central role in healthy nervous system function and hormone balance. Since in some cases stress and tension may hinder conception, it is wise to develop a nutritional regimen that nourishes the nervous system. Many people claim they feel less stressed when they faithfully take their "B's."

The B vitamins also play a key role in hormone balance. A deficiency of B vitamins can create an excess of estrogen in the system and, conversely, an excess of estrogen can create a B vitamin deficiency. The B vitamins are found mostly in whole grains, and most are lost in processing. Evidence also suggests that B vitamins are lost to refined sugar, stress, caffeine, alcohol and other drugs.

Vitamin A

Although it is most widely recognized for its connection to healthy vision—especially night vision—many scientists have found a link between vitamin A and healthy sperm production.[55]

In one study, researchers fed a group of rats a vitamin-A deficient diet from the time they were three weeks old until they were about four months old. They developed degeneration of and loss of sperm cells. Within six weeks of vitamin A treatment new sperm appeared.[56]

Department of Agriculture studies conducted over a 30-year time span found that vitamin A is one of the four major nutrients Americans are not getting enough of. The other three are vitamin C, calcium and iron.

Megadoses of vitamin A were the subject of a great deal of negative publicity several years ago, because megadoses of this vitamin can be toxic. Unlike water-soluble vitamins, which the body can eliminate when it has more than it needs, vitamin A is stored in the liver and can build up to the point of toxicity.

The best source of vitamin A is its precursor, beta carotene, the substance from which the body can manufacture vitamin A as needed. Supplements containing beta carotene can be purchased from a natural foods store.

The ancient Egyptians prescribed cooked liver as a cure for some eye disorders. Liver just happens to be high in vitamin A. Another excellent source of vitamin A is fish liver oils, available at health food stores.

Do not take more than 25,000 IU of vitamin A daily without consulting a health professional.

Food Sources of Beta Carotene

Apricots, asparagus, broccoli, cantaloupe, carrots, cherries, cress, dandelion greens, kale, mangoes, peaches, peas, romaine lettuce, sweet potatoes, spinach, tomatoes, winter squash.

Selenium

Studies have shown that populations living in areas with soil rich in selenium demonstrate higher birth rates. Although extensive studies on this mineral haven't been conducted, early reports indicate a connection between selenium and sperm production. At least half of the selenium in the male body is found in the semen. Infertility is observed in animals with selenium deficiencies. Selenium may be as important as zinc for the production of healthy sperm.[57]

Researchers discovered that a lower conception rate in a test group of young animals was directly related to selenium deficiency.[58] Selenium-vitamin E combination has been used to overcome infertility in animals.

The RDA (Recommended Daily Allowance) for selenium is 50 to 200 micrograms. The average diet contains 20 to 60 micrograms, which clearly leaves room for supplementation.

Symptoms of selenium deficiency include cardiovascular disease, high blood pressure, arthritis, cataracts, dermatitis, sexual dysfunction and infertility.[59] Of course, since these are symptoms of many other deficiencies it would be difficult to determine whether you have a selenium deficiency or not. Making sure your dietary intake at least meets the RDA is the best course of action.

Food Sources of Selenium

Whole grains, eggs.

Calcium-Vitamin D

Experts have long known that a vitamin D deficiency in test animals reduces fertility by as much as 75 percent. University of Wisconsin experts decided to determine whether vitamin D or calcium would cure vitamin-D induced infertility.

Researchers divided infertile male rats into two test groups. One vitamin-D-deficient group was treated with a vitamin D supplement. Another group was given extra calcium. Fertility was restored in both groups, suggesting that vitamin D affects fertility by influencing calcium metabolism in reproductive tissues.

Researchers concluded that if the test results can be applied to men, at least 4,000 IU of vitamin D should be consumed daily to ensure normal fertility.[60]

Food Sources of Calcium

Dairy products, broccoli, kale, collards, tofu.

Food Sources of Vitamin D

Eggs, butter.

SUMMARY OF VITAMINS, MINERALS AND FERTILITY

Because the vitamin-mineral-fertility connection is still in its infant stages of research, new developments are sure to break. Until we know more, let common sense be your guide. The best place to get needed nutrients is from a healthy diet focused on foods in their whole state, but many foods are nutrient-deficient so supplementation may be needed.

Perhaps scientists are discovering that certain nutrients enhance fertility because these nutrients are lacking in the highly processed diet. If the nutrients had originally been present in the diet, fertility problems may have never been present in the first place.

Finally, vitamins and minerals are not miracle drugs, but are food substances necessary for the normal functioning of the human body. As such, they take time to work. If you want a quick, druglike fix, you probably won't get one from nutrients because rebalancing the body takes time. But when certain nutrients are lacking in the human diet, supplementation can often lead to impressive results.

4 ___ The Wonderful World of Herbs

Even before the days of Lydia Pinkham's herbal female tonic formula in the late 1800s, which claimed to have "a baby in every bottle," women have used herbs for their unique needs. The herbal tradition is thousands of years old, and only for the past several decades has it been overshadowed by the modern medical revolution—at least in America.

A good thing is bound to endure. Herbs are getting more and more attention these days. They're no longer a fad for a few holdouts from the '60s. Herbs are taking hold of mainstream America, and even the mainstream media has taken notice. I was forced to take notice because I've heard so many herb success stories from completely honest people. These aren't miracle stories; they're stories of people who got to the roots of their problems and took the time to properly strengthen the body nutritionally, thereby setting in action the body's own healing mechanisms.

Those who haven't heard a lot about herbs sometimes have the mistaken impression that they belong in the same category as witchcraft and black cats. Unfortunately, herbs have gotten a bum rap the past few decades, at least in the United States. That's because in the rapture of modern medicine, we've forgotten our medicinal roots (no pun intended).

Despite their falling into the sidelight for the past 50 decades or so, herbs have withstood the test of time. Eighty percent of the world's population still uses herbs as the main form of medicine. Those herbs that don't furnish the benefits they're claimed to furnish probably would have fallen by the wayside a long time ago. Interestingly, often one herb is used for the same conditions in countries throughout the world, by cultures that have had no evidence of contact with each other. Is this coincidence, or evidence that herbs really work? Despite the fact that much of our knowledge about herbs is anecdotal, science is catching up and verifying many of those claims made by the folk of yesteryear.

Why don't the powers that be conduct more studies on the benefits of herbs? The answer is mostly a matter of economics. Herbs are naturally occurring substances, and naturally occurring substances cannot be patented. Because it can take millions of dollars to research a plant extensively enough to prove that it has medicinal benefits—the procedure necessary to receive FDA approval to make medicinal claims for an herb—and the plant itself cannot be patented, researchers could never charge the exorbitant fees to market an herb that would be necessary to recap their research dollars. So generally, they pursue substances they can patent—especially in the United States. Patentability is one of the main reasons scientists make synthetic versions of plant substances.

Still, more than half of our modern medicines are plant-based. Aspirin, for example, is based on salicylic acid, which is found in white willow bark. One of the most recent plant-drug discoveries is taxol, from the bark of the Pacific yew tree in the northwestern United States, which shows great promise in the treatment of ovarian and breast cancer. Cascara sagrada, the bark of a tree which grows in the Northwest, is used extensively in the pharmaceutical industry in laxative preparations. Aloe vera is one of the better known healing plants. It soothes burns on contact and speeds the healing process.

The fact that plants have chemical compounds which can work wonders on the human body is indisputable. The current effort on the part of the FDA to have some herbs and vitamins available only by prescription is point-blank evidence that they work. It is also evidence that the established medical field feels threatened by the growing number of people turning to natural health care, despite claims that it is "only trying to protect us"—from natural substances that have been freely used for thousands of years?

Whole herbs have many benefits not found in their synthetically isolated compounds. Naturalists believe when you isolate medicinal compounds from a plant, you lose the balancing qualities of the plant's other compounds which prevent side-effects. Hence, drugs almost always have side effects, whereas herbs rarely do. Drugs often create serious side-effects and even death. Herbs, when used with a little intelligence and common sense, rarely have side-effects. The amount of reputable literature available on herbs makes their safe use almost guaranteed.

Despite their general lack of support by the American scientific and medical communities, herbs are still the main form of health care around the world. They can play an important role in cleansing and balancing the body—not because they have magical powers, but because they have chemical components from natural sources readily assimable by the body. They can furnish elements missing in the everyday diet. They can also work wonders on the human body that we haven't yet explained scientifically.

Herbs have been used for fertility problems for thousands of years. A classic case is found in the Bible, with the story of Rachel and Leah. Rachel tried for years to conceive, and felt great despair when she continued to be unsuccessful. She moaned to her husband, "Give me children, or else I die!" She finally ate mandrakes, and ended up conceiving (Genesis 30). Whether you believe the story or not, it clearly illustrates the historical reputation of certain herbs for promoting fertility.

Modern miracles exist, too. Bente (Bent'-uh), a good friend of mine from Norway, suffered from severe endometriosis throughout her late twenties and early thirties. At age 31 she started to take prescribed birth control pills in an effort to control the problem. She ended up undergoing four surgeries to remove adhesions and endometriosis. She often suffered from extreme fatigue and depression and severe pain, even after the surgeries. Fed up with traditional medicine, she sought out natural alternatives. (This is the point many people reach before they discover the wonders of natural health care.)

Bente was 33 by the time she started on an herbal program, and wanted very much to get married. Her doctor doubted that she would ever have children. Not only was she getting a late start, but also her four surgeries left her with a great deal of scar tissue on her reproductive organs. After faithfully using the herbs for several months, she went back to her gynecologist. He examined her and told her she'd never looked better.

Not only was her health better, but her outward appearance improved as well. Her complexion brightened; her eyes sparkled. After she turned to natural alternatives, she looked better than I'd ever seen her. It was as if she finally had hope. I noticed the difference in her countenance even before she told me she was using herbs.

Her story had a very happy ending. Bente married at age 33 and, much to my surprise, ended up with a honeymoon baby! I hate to admit it, but I was disappointed to not have a partner in my infertile misery! There are no scientific tests to prove that herbs had anything to do with her success story, but she believes with all her heart they did and shares her story with everyone she can. Her doctor said it was a miracle.

Bente's program, which she followed faithfully for the 10 months before she married, consisted of the following:

- an herbal combination rich in dong quai
- vitamin B6
- zinc
- liquid chlorophyll
- evening primrose oil (recently banned because of insufficient evidence for its benefits, despite its great record of success in female problems and no evidence that it has any harmful effects; black currant oil is a good substitute)

For two months she ate a completely vegetarian diet. "Meats like beef and pork don't go well with female problems," Bente says.

In order to reap the full benefits of herbs, would-be parents should cleanse the body and focus on a diet of wholesome foods. You can't expect to drink a six-pack of cola per day, indulge in liquor, consume mostly highly processed foods and still experience the full benefits of herbs.

Couples trying to get their bodies in optimal health would do well to begin by cleansing the colon with daily use of psyllium fiber (the ingredient in Metamucil) or cascara sagrada, both non-addictive helps for cleansing the colon. Natural health advocates believe when the colon is not properly eliminating waste matter, toxins back up and enter the bloodstream, causing all kinds of unhealthy conditions. Before the advent of modern medicine, this theory (autointoxication=self-poisoning) was widely accepted and enemas were given for many health concerns. My mother still remembers the practice. For more information about cleansing, see Appendix A.

Because the liver plays such a key role in hormone balance, women may benefit from herbal combinations with nutrients targetted at the liver in addition to those for balancing the hormones. Be sure to use a reputable herb source.

The following herbs can be purchased separately or in combinations specifically targetted to nourish male or female reproductive systems.

FOR WOMEN
Dong Quai

This herb, often called the Queen of the Female Herbs, has been used for thousands of years by women in China to nourish and balance the reproductive system. It comes from the root of the *angelica sinensis* plant, grown in certain Chinese provinces. The name means "compelled to return," signifying a woman returning to her normal female functions. Some say the name connotes a woman's reverting to her husband, with implied fertility virtues.

Chinese women use dong quai for menstrual period regulation. Many claim it nourishes the blood and promotes the growth of the womb. Research has shown that it helps in menopause and soothes cramps. It is being used by European medical doctors for painful menstruation, excessive bleeding and suppressed menstruation. Many herbalists claim it dissolves blood clots and opens blocked passageways in the body.

Modern science has verified that dong quai is rich in vitamin E, cobalt and iron. It is believed to be nourishing to female glands for that and other reasons.

For overall balance and the health of the reproductive system, dong quai is an excellent herb to use. The Chinese say it takes three months of regular use to notice the herb's benefits.

Red Raspberry

Red raspberry leaves also rank high on the list of herbal remedies for women. This herb is rich in iron and is highly recommended during pregnancy. It has also been used for menstrual discomforts with great success. While red raspberry has no fertility claims attached to its use, women have used it for centuries to nourish and strengthen the female system.

Red raspberry leaves contain significant amounts of vitamin C, as well as vitamins A, B-complex, D, E, iron, phosphorus, manganese and calcium.

Black Cohosh

Black cohosh is native to the Eastern forests of the United States and Canada, and was used extensively by Native Americans.

It is traditionally used as a hormone-balancing herb, and in female complaints such as dysmenorrhea and amenorrhea. This herb should be taken in small amounts. Any you purchase from a reputable source will have a recommended daily dosage printed on the label.

Many women take it as an estrogen supplement, though no proven estrogenic qualities have been found in it.

Alfalfa

Alfalfa, which grows abundantly in the wild and is cultivated extensively for animal food, is best known as an overall nutritive herb, rich in trace minerals needed by the glandular system of the body. Alfalfa roots grow deep, picking up minerals that may not be found in the top layers of soil. Alfalfa contains high amounts of beta carotene, the precursor to vitamin A. It also helps to purify the blood, partially due to its high chlorophyll content. Using alfalfa is a good way to supply extra nutrients which may be missing from your diet—nutrients necessary for the health of the glandular system.

Kelp

Like alfalfa, kelp is rich in trace minerals. Both herbs are usually included in herbal formulas targetted to nourishing the glands. Kelp is native to the Pacific coast, although other related species of seaweed are native to the Atlantic coast. Herbalists sometimes use kelp as a blood purifier. It contains significant amounts of iodine, calcium and potassium. Because of its iodine content, kelp as a nutritional supplement is helpful for those with first-generation hypothyroid (underactive thyroid), a common cause of miscarriage.

Ho Shou Wu

According to Chinese folk medicine, ho shou wu enhances fertility. Scientists have put that claim to the test. Daniel Mowrey, Ph.D., summarizes a scientific study reported by the U.S. Herbal Delegation. To directly quote from the study, "In aminals, extracts of this plant show antitumor activity, as well as antiprogestation activity, sedative effects, and antipyretic effects." In other words, in animals ho shou wu extract demonstrated beneficial effects on fertility and other female functions involving ovulation and corpus luteum formation.[61]

False Unicorn

False unicorn grows in moist regions in the eastern third of the United States. Herbalists use it as a uterine tonic, diuretic, and menstrual pain tonic. Historically, many herbalists have recommended it for ovarian pain and dysfunctions of the ovaries. The root part of the plant is used. Of all the herbs, false unicorn has one of the strongest reputations for promoting fertility. Although this has not been scientifically verified (no studies of this nature have been conducted), there is a great deal of anecdotal evidence in its favor.

Dr. Christopher, a famous herbalist, recommended false unicorn with other herbs and nutrients for couples having difficulty conceiving. He reported great success.

Damiana

Damiana is a highly aromatic shrub which grows in the desert regions of the southwest United States and Mexico. Women in Mexico use it for female problems. Some herbalists recommend it for increasing fertility in both sexes and for increasing sexual desire, although this is a traditional use and has not been scientifically verified. It is a common ingredient in both male and female tonic formulas. You'll recognize the word "aphrodisiac" in its Latin name, *turnera aphrodisiaca*.

Yams

A professor at the University of Ibadan in Nigeria conducted studies on the native Yoruba tribe, who have one of the highest rate of twin births in the world. The professor found that their diet contained large amounts of yams (sweet potatoes).

Yams have long been reputed to help in infertility, but science is only recently finding evidence to back this long-held belief. Yams contain steroidlike compounds which can be easily converted into sex hormones. They are sometimes used as the raw material for making contraceptives.

The compounds trigger the release of FSH, which stimulates the ovaries to release an egg. In this case high yam consumption seems to stimulate the release of more than one egg each month. Women in the Yoruba tribe have high levels of FSH.

This news was reported in *Alternatives*, July 1989. The author added that researchers feel one-half cup of sweet potatoes daily might increase one's chance of having twins.[62] For the infertile couple, it may increase your chance of having one child!

Blessed Thistle

This herb is native to Asia and the Mediterranean area. The name comes from the belief centuries ago that this plant was a cure-all.

Blessed thistle is used in many herbal combinations as a hormone-balancing aid and in overcoming menstrual problems. Although it does not have the specific reputation for increasing fertility, it may be useful for general female problems.

Liquid Chlorophyll

Chlorophyll, the green pigment found in plants, is an excellent body cleanser and is available in liquid form through health food stores and independent herb distributors. It has the reputation of regulating menstruation, helping to purify the liver, building the blood and having many other beneficial effects on the body. Some natural health enthusiasts call it "liquid sunshine." It makes an excellent dietary supplement for a program of overall health and cleansing.

Liquid chlorophyll of the health food store variety comes from alfalfa plants.

FOR MEN

The herbs beneficial for women are generally beneficial for men as well. However, a few herbs do receive more attention for their effects on the male reproductive system. Bee pollen, listed in this section, is an excellent nutritional supplement for both men and women.

Siberian Ginseng

Many forms of ginseng grow around the world—American ginseng, Panax ginseng, Korean ginseng and Siberian ginseng. Ginseng has become one of the most studied herbs of all time. Researchers in the former Soviet Union have done the most research on Siberian ginseng, a close relative of Panax ginseng.

Many of Siberian ginseng's healthful properties have been scientifically verified. It is widely used by people around the world as a general tonic, and is almost always a main ingredient in male tonics. Many believe that it has aphrodisiac properties, enhancing and increasing male sexual function. It can also be used by women to aid in balancing the glandular system and helping to promote a general state of good health.

Studies done in the animal husbandry industry have shown that Siberian ginseng has pronounced effects on the reproductive system. "In comparison with controls, more milk was made by cows, more honey by bees, and minks produced more living young." In the minks' case, according to a 1988 article in *Nutrition News*, "the number of sterile females was lowered and stillborn births were reduced by 50 percent." Bulls given Siberian ginseng also showed increased virility.[63]

According to the *Nutrition News* article, experiments in China showed that ginseng affects the production of LH, the lutenizing hormone, which influences the menstrual cycle and stimulates testosterone production in men.

Sarsaparilla

Sarsaparilla is a tropical plant native to Central and South America. The bitter root is used in herbology. The plant is widely used commercially as a flavoring and foaming agent in foods such as root beer. You might recognize the name of this plant as a familiar soda drink.

In natural health circles sarsaparilla is considered both a male and a female tonic. Natives of the Far East, New Guinea and Central America use it as an aphrodisiac. Claims that it contains the hormones testosterone, progesterone and cortin were made by Professor Russel E. Marker and Dr. Aval Rohrmon.[64] Those claims have been proven neither false nor true. One Hungarian researcher succeeded in synthetically producing testosterone from a component in sarsaparilla.[65]

Sarsaparilla has been scientifically proven to contain two substances called sarsapogenin and smilagenen, which are used in the production of synthetic steroids.[66] Hence, its reputation as a male and female tonic appears to hold some weight.

Saw Palmetto

Native to the coastal areas of Florida and Texas, the saw palmetto plant has a long history of use as food by the native Indians of the region. The part of the plant most often used in herbology is the berries.

Clinical trials conducted with saw palmetto showed that the fruit helps reduce symptoms of BPH, a condition in which the prostate enlarges and causes restriction of the urinary tract. The FDA would not allow any claims to be made for the fruit because BPH is not a self-limiting condition, and consumers might diagnose and prescribe their own treatment. The bottom line: saw palmetto berries were shown to have a positive effect on prostate function, but the FDA will not allow health foods businesses to make such claims.[67]

Saw palmetto has also been shown to have estrogenic compounds. Traditionally, the herb has been used as a male tonic, aphrodisiac, and general glandular nourisher.

Pumpkin Seed

Pumpkin seeds are rich in zinc, a nutrient important to the healthy functioning of the male reproductive system. You can purchase them in powdered, encapsulated form at most health food stores.

Bee Pollen

Although bee pollen is not an herb, it does come from flowers. Pollen is produced by the male part of flowering plants. Bees carry the pollen from flower to flower, an action which cross-pollinates and fertilizes seeds. The bees carry some of the pollen on their back legs to the hive, where they use it for food.

The Hunzas, who live in the Himalayan Mountains, and the Caucasus people of Russia—both renowned for their health and longevity—eat above-average quantities of bee pollen and raw honey. Many athletes and other health-conscious individuals consume bee pollen as an energy-promoting food supplement. Even Ronald Reagan, former United

States president, reportedly uses bee pollen to increase his overall health and stamina.

Bee pollen is considered a complete food. It contains all the vitamins and minerals necessary for survival. It also contains the 10 essential amino acids necessary to make a complete protein, as well as enzymes and coenzymes. Among the many health benefits of pollen are claims that it balances glandular activity and increases fertility in some cases.

According to one report, 40 men in infertile marriages where sperm deficiency was the cause of infertility took supplementary bee pollen. It proved to solve the problem. After taking bee pollen the men reported improved health in general, an increase in sexual activity and improved sperm production.[68]

In a study conducted by Bogdan Tekavcic, M.D., chief of a gynecolgical center in Yugoslavia, bee pollen corrected some menstrual problems. Half of a group of women with menstrual complaints were given bee pollen with royal jelly, and the other half were given a placebo. Almost all the women on the royal jelly-pollen regimen showed improvement or a disappearance of their menstrual problems, whereas the placebo group showed little change.[69]

If you have plant or pollen allergies, you might be allergic to bee pollen. On the other hand, bee pollen helps some people overcome allergies. Ask a health professional for advice.

Damiana
(see under "For Women")

COMBINATIONS

For the Liver

Hormone balance is dependent largely upon a properly functioning liver. Herb formulas for supporting the liver usually contain various combinations of some of the following herbs—red beet root, dandelion, parsley, horsetail, liverwort, black cohosh, birth, blessed thistle, angelica, chamomile, gentian, golden seal, barberry, ginger, cramp bark, fennel seed, peppermint, wild yam, and catnip.

For Female Problems

Some believe combinations work better than single herbs. Look for combinations containing the following herbs—red raspberry, dong quai, ginger, licorice, black cohosh, queen of the meadow, blessed thistle, marshmallow, golden seal, capsicum, false unicorn, cramp bark, and squaw vine.

Chinese Combinations

Chinese herbal combinations for fertility problems often focus on purifying the blood, strengthening the liver, enhancing immunity and balancing the hormones. Herbs commonly included in such formulas include dong quai, Panax ginseng, ho shou wu, rehmannia, astragalus, ganoderma, and peony root.

For the Glands

The glands depend upon a good supply of trace minerals. Good gland-nourishing formulas are based on herbs rich in minerals such as kelp, dandelion, Irish moss, hops, capsicum, and parsley.

For the untimid—organotherapy: Glandulars, or dehydrated, dessicated animal glands, can also be used to support human glandular activity. The thought may seem shocking to the 20th century mind, but animal products have been used in health care for centuries. For instance, dessicated animal thyroid has been used for thyroid problems for at least 100 years, and is still prescribed by doctors today.

The theory behind glandulars is that the dried animal glands still contain the proteins, hormones and other substances that were active in the live animal. These same substances stimulate activity in the human glands, helping them return to normalcy.

For Male Vitality

Look for combinations containing some of the following herbs—Siberian ginseng, echinacea, saw palmetto, damiana, sarsaparilla, garlic, and capsicum.

Blood Purifiers

Proper hormone balance and overall health depends upon healthy blood. Blood purifiers, or spring tonics, were popular before the advent of modern medicine. A good blood-purifying combination should feature herbs such as chapparal, pau d'arco, red clover, dandelion, cascara sagrada, red clover, and burdock.

SUMMARY ON HERBS

Mankind has used herbs for medicinal reasons at least since the beginning of recorded history. Modern science is verifying the significant manner in which herbs can help the body heal itself. Herbs can often be very effective in balancing the body and enhancing fertility.

Learning about and using herbs can also be a great adventure. As you become familiar with the herbs in this section, why not expand your knowledge to include others? You'll be participating in a rich tradition thousands of years old.

For even more fun, you can learn about the herbs that grow in your particular area of the country, or grow your own. Learning how to cultivate, dry and store herbs can open up a whole new hobby for you.

5 —————— A Hodgepodge of Helpful Hints

People love to give infertile couples advice. "Stand on your head"; "Go on a vacation,"; "Just relax,"; "Take vitamin E," and "Stop thinking about it," are a few of the helpful hints I've heard. While some helpful hints are less than helpful, some actually do get results. In this chapter I've compiled all the helpful hints with at least some substance behind them.

Stand on Your Head

As one doctor put it, "Make gravity work for you." A co-worker of mine knew the couple who heard this advice. They'd been trying for two years to get pregnant. When the girl stood on her head after intercourse, she conceived.

You'll surely laugh at the thought of standing on your head after intercourse, and your husband is sure to laugh a bit too, but another woman I work with told me she knows of two couples who tried it and found it worked after a couple cycles. Perhaps it was coincidence—but maybe not.

Actually, it makes sense. You'll give your husband's sperm much more chance to make its way to your egg by using the laws of gravity in your favor. Many doctors will laugh at this recommendation, but many also suggest trying it. You have nothing to lose.

If you don't want to get quite so drastic, you can lie on your back and elevate your hips with a pillow—or try anything else that elevates your hips.

Abstinence Makes the Seeds Grow Stronger

Actually, it makes the sperm count grow stronger. Many doctors recommend that a couple trying to get pregnant abstain for several days before the wife's fertile period to increase sperm count. One recommendation is to abstain for the first two or three days after menstruation ends.

One good friend of mine who had been trying to get pregnant for over a year made her husband abstain for about a week before her fertile time (a difficult task for him) and she elevated her hips after intercourse. She conceived that time around, and has since given birth to a healthy baby girl!

Cool Down

Men, don't hang out in hot tubs, saunas, hot baths, steam baths, and under electric blankets, which are known as notorious sperm killers. Anything which leads to a constant elevation in scrotal temperature should be avoided.

Give Up on Your Marathon Races

Many women who exercise strenuously stop having their periods. If this is the case for you, lighten up on the exercise for awhile and give your body a chance to return to normal.

Too much exercise can reduce body fat below the level needed for a pregnancy to occur. If a woman's body fat falls below a certain percentage, estrogen production tapers off, ovulation can cease and infertility may result. The stress involved in strenuous exercise may also be a culprit.

Several studies have shown that decreased ovarian function is one of the body's first responses to decreased caloric intake.[70]

Don't Wear Your Jeans a Little Bit Tighter

"I'm wearing my jeans a little bit tighter" sings the country star. But if your husband is singing this song, you might want to discourage him. Too-tight jeans can keep the scrotal sac too close to the body, making it too warm and resulting in lethargic sperm. The sperm rests away from the body for a reason: to keep it cooler.

Researchers think the lowering sperm count of today's male is partly due to the popularity of tight-fitting underwear which has become popular since the 1950s. A study at the University of Nebraska Medical Center by a Dr. Patrick Friman showed that men who wore jockey-style underwear had a lower sperm count than men who wore loose boxer-type shorts—by as many as 12 million per milliliter.[71]

Baking Soda Douche

Use a baking soda douche before intercourse if you suspect your vagina is too acidic, as it may be killing too many sperm. Use one or two tablespoons soda to one quart water.

Don't Use Lubricating Jelly Before Intercourse

Lubricating jelly has never been proven to interfere with conception, but many doctors recommend not using it to maximize your chance of conceiving. It may make getting around more difficult for the sperm.

Some doctors now recommend that couples trying to conceive use egg white warmed to room temperature for lubrication during a woman's fertile time, if necessary. The thought may shock you, but doctors claim the consistency is more like a woman's own cervical mucus and rich in protein, making sperm passage much easier in the egg white. The tip is offered by Andrew Toledo, M.D., fertility specialist at Emory University.[72]

You only need to use the egg white during your fertile times; at other times of the month, use whatever you prefer.

Make Love in the Missionary Position

This means, of course, with the man on top. Make sure ejaculation occurs deep within the vagina, so sperm is deposited close to the cervix. This may give the sperm a greater chance to meet an egg.

Know Your Fertile Time

No matter how hard you try, if intercourse does not occur during your fertile period, you won't get pregnant. There are several clues your body can give to show you it's in the fertile period of your cycle. One is an increased mucus discharge or wetness anywhere from 10 to 14 days from the start of your last period. Another is a dull ache in one of your ovaries around ovulation time, a phenomenon known as Mittelschmertz.

Another is a rise in body temperature during ovulation time of at least .8 degree and as much as 1.5 degrees which stays higher until menstruation begins. If pregnancy occurs, the temperature remains higher throughout pregnancy. To use the temperature method of determining whether ovulation occurs, the temperature must be taken every day before getting out of bed, first thing upon awakening. However, this method is not always accurate.

If you're on a 28-day cycle, ovulation will usually occur 14 days after the beginning of your last cycle.

Try Some Cough Syrup

Oral decongestants can also play the role of thinning too-thick cervical mucus, which sometimes acts like a natural diaphragm. Take the syrup orally, of course!

Husbands: Wear a Condom for a Couple Months

Women who develop antibodies to their partner's sperm may overcome the problem if their man wears a condom for several months during intercourse. This gives the body time to decrease its production of antibodies, so the next time sperm is introduced the antibodies won't overreact.

Go on a Vacation

Doctors hate to read "rubbish" like this, but anecdotal evidence does show that some couples conceive during vacations and other relaxing occasions, when their minds are not on temperature charts, timing and the other mechanics of conception.

One woman tried for years to conceive, using the standard temperature charts and timing methods. She went on a vacation, and at a time seemingly impossible, long after ovulation should have occured, she conceived. There may be something to it!

Lose a Few Pounds

Just as being underweight can affect ovulation, so can being overweight. In fact, being overweight can double a woman's chances of being infertile. If you have a weight problem and are having trouble conceiving, losing a few pounds may increase your chances of pregnancy.

Fat cells help manufacture estrogen, so an overproduction of estrogen may contribute to infertility in overweight women.

SUMMARY ON HELPFUL HINTS

If nothing else, by trying the suggestions in this chapter you'll get a vacation, your husband will get some new boxer shorts, and you'll both have some cough syrup on hand for the next flu outbreak.

6 ___ The Emotional Factor

Jane (not her real name) tried for three years to get pregnant. She visited her doctor and he conducted all of the tests possible to determine a cause for her infertility. She took fertility drugs for a month but stopped because she couldn't afford them. She finally decided to give up the idea of ever having a baby and stopped thinking about it. She stopped all forms of treatment—and conceived.

Jane's story is not unusual. Many couples conceive when they simply stop thinking about getting pregnant or experience a general improvement in their life satisfaction—which suggests that the mind-body-fertility connection is in operation.

Nothing is more frustrating for an infertile couple than when well-meaning but uninformed friends and relatives chirp, "Just relax—it'll happen." Some people will even tell you the problem is all in your head. In writing this chapter, I'm in no way trying to trivialize infertility or blame it on psychology. In most cases, an organic cause exists for the inability to get pregnant. However, in a few cases psychological barriers can, for whatever reason, prevent conception. This chapter will explore these possible barriers and offer solutions.

The Post-Adoption Syndrome

If psychological factors play no part in the ability to conceive, why is it that so many couples struggle for years to have children, adopt, and then get pregnant? Every infertile couple has probably heard more conception-after-adoption stories than they cared to hear. No one would recommend adopting so you'll get pregnant, and not every couple that adopts does get pregnant afterwards. Still, the stories can't help but suggest there's some kind of psychological connection between adoption and subsequent conception.

Many doctors deny any correlation between adoption and pregnancy, claiming the same percentage of infertile couples conceive who don't adopt as those who do adopt. Which side you choose to believe is up to you.

While waiting for a haircut one day I read a story in a popular women's magazine about a woman who had tried for years to get pregnant. She'd had surgeries on her ovaries (ovarian wedges) and doctors said her ovaries were so damaged she'd never have children. Deciding that the door to having their own children had been closed, she and her husband adopted several children, brothers and sisters, all at one time. Two months later, she was pregnant—with twins.

Perhaps once couples adopt and get their mind off having a child, their bodies finally relax and set in motion the forces needed for conception.

I recently listened to a story of a couple in which the husband was told because of his poor sperm, they'd probably never conceive. Within months after the doctor said they'd never conceive, the wife got pregnant. Perhaps hearing that they'd never have children removed the pressure and actually led to the conception.

David J. Gyertson, guest host of the television show the *700 Club* and president of Regent University in Virginia Beach, Virginia, shared the story of he and his wife's six-year struggle to have children. Doctors finally told him his sperm count was so low as to make him functionally sterile. Shortly afterwards, without medical intervention, his wife conceived. He chalks it up to a miracle.

There are many theories as to why couples conceive after adoptions and doctor write-offs, but one deserving further exploration is the emotional factor. Doctors, spiritual leaders, mystics and others have puzzled over the mind/body connection for thousands of years. Scientists are only recently discovering how strong this connection is.

Can Good Thoughts Heal the Body?

Dr. Bernie Siegel, noted medical doctor, lecturer and author, believes so. In 1978 Dr. Siegel started a form of group therapy for terminal cancer patients called "Exceptional Cancer Patients." Siegel believes the connection between mind and body is so strong that by the year 2000 it will be accepted as a scientific fact.

He has many examples to back his belief. In a lecture in Salt Lake City, Utah, Siegel shared the story of a lawyer who had a brain tumor, and left his practice to take up what he'd always wanted to do: play the violin. Within a year, there was no sign of a brain tumor.

According to Siegel, hope is a kind of medicine. Feelings of discouragement and despair release certain chemicals into the body, while positive feelings and hope release another. The bad chemicals break down body tissues, while the good chemicals repair them. Siegel holds that our thoughts affect our immune system.

Siegel says there's a lot more to medicine than pills, surgeries and laboratories. Because of the unexplained cures he's witnessed in his many years of practice, he's come to the conclusion that a person's state of mind affects the state of his or her body. Siegel believes there are no incurable diseases, only incurable people. "Those who are able to love and hope, have peace of mind and faith send their bodies a 'live' message, while those who are constantly depressed, fearful, despairing and in conflict and do nothing about it give their bodies a 'die' message."[73]

While thinking positive thoughts will not guarantee you a child, an attitude of hope may offer you better health and peace of mind—which may, in turn, lead to a pregnancy.

The body is designed to heal itself. When you cut a finger, blood comes rushing to the surface and coagulates as a healing mechanism. Tissues renew themselves continuously. Symptoms are manifestations that the body is trying to heal itself. A positive outlook combined with the nutritional principles in this book can create the state of physical and mental health you need to conceive.

Chiropractor George Goodheart stated, "The human body has a remarkable built-in healing mechanism; it is constructed and programmed in such a way that it can heal itself. In chiropractic we speak of an innate intelligence or physiological homeostasis that automatically strives to restore equilibrium in the body when an imbalance occurs in any of its many complex systems. This innate intelligence is the common basis for all healing. People are healed by many different kinds of healers and systems because the real healer is within. The various healing modalities are merely different ways of activating that inner healer."

Scientifically Speaking

Psychoneuroendocrinology is the study of the relationship between emotions, the nervous system and the endocrine (hormone) system. Scientists have verified that emotions definitely affect the body's delicately balanced hormone functions.

They've discovered that depression, stress and other forms of psychological trauma can set off chemical processes in the body that interfere with ovulation. Researchers discovered that in one group of women who failed to ovulate, a high proportion of them had experienced different forms of psychological trauma before or around the time of puberty.

Polycystic ovary disease and hyperprolactinemia (elevated prolactin in the blood) have both been linked to hormone imbalances caused by stress in some cases. The fact that prolonged stress and anxiety can lead to elevated prolactin is no longer a theory, but is a proven fact. And when one hormone is thrown out of balance, such as prolactin, other imbalances sometimes follow in a chain reaction.

Some analytic psychiatrists suggest that an unconscious psychological defense mechanism protects women who fear motherhood against conception by affecting the physical processes of reproduction. Such ideas are merely speculation, but they offer an intriguing theory for unexplained infertility.

According to fertility expert Dr. Machelle M. Siebel, "It has been known since ancient times that a relationship exists between the menstrual cycle and the psyche. The study of the emotional aspects of infertility is rapidly moving from considerations of psychological presets, psychic trauma, and developmental influences to investigating the production, reception and effects of transmitter amines in brain centers associated with emotions and reproduction."[74] All of this is a scientific way of saying emotions can significantly affect the chemical processes involved in reproduction.

One of the doctors I visited about fertility early in my marriage told me his belief that when a woman is overly anxious about becoming pregnant, the fallopian tubes can spasm and interfere with the passage of sperm.

My doctor wasn't the only one to recognize the effect anxiety can have on the reproductive system. According to medical doctor John J. Stangel, "Stress can affect the coordinated movement of the fallopian tubes that allow the egg to be transported in one direction and the sperm in another. Proper tubal movement, pickup of the egg, and its movement toward the uterus may be hampered, thus leading to infertility."[75]

Emotional factors can also supress oogenesis, reduce the fertility of the ovum, and alter cervical secretions. One research team discovered that stress can actually result in the production of cervical secretions that interefere with sperm migration, a situation which often reverses when the emotional stress is resolved.[76]

Women aren't the only ones adversely affected by stress. A man's sperm count and motility can be negatively affected as well. One expert reports:

> Psychic stress, especially conflicts over fatherhood, may, for example, produce enzymatic changes in the sperm. Sperm quantity and motility may be normal, but, if one or more enzymatic systems are missing as a result of faulty protein synthesis, the genetic organizier material necessary for normal fertilizing power will not be present. It is recognized that stress disrupts nucleoprotein metabolism and interferes with the sperm's capacity to fertilize. Yet, scant attention has been paid to these kinds of infertility questions.[77]

Several true-life experiences bear this statement out. In one case, a man's sperm count dropped drastically after an auto accident in which he was not injured. His count remained low for four months, after which it returned to the level it was prior to the accident.[78] In other studies, severe and progressive deficiencies in sperm production were discovered in prisoners who were sentenced with the death penalty but had to wait a long time before the execution was carried out.[79]

A research team by the name of Kleegman and Kaufman in 1966 discovered that improving a group of infertile men's psychological state also improved their sperm count. They observed that sperm improvement is often effected by a job change which reduces tension, improves the subject's economic status, and increases overall satisfaction with life. Another evidence that psychological factors play a role in the production of sperm is the phenomenon that production often improves following the use of a placebo.

One doctor even went so far as to develop a personality profile of the average infertile male. Society tends to relate the macho-man image with virility, but Dr. D.H. Hellhammer found otherwise.

The West German doctor used personality questionnaires to classify the male partner in 117 infertile couples. He matched the data with how potent each man's sperm was. The result? The more aggressive, demanding men produced sperm that were less active and fewer in number.

Dr. Hellhammer used for his control group fertile husbands, among them men who were neurotic, depressed and anxious. The factor that seemed to play a role in reproductive success was lack of stress. Aggressive men, concluded the doctor, are under more internal stress than balanced men because they feel a constant need to fight against or change their external circumstances.[80]

Stress can create almost any reproductive problem, as evidenced by the following list:

Reproductive Problems Which Have Been Linked to Stress[81]

Impotence	Dyspareunia	Vaginismus
Oligospermia	Azoospermia	Deficient sperm motility
Deficient sperm form	Retrograde ejaculation	Premature ejaculation
Egg abnormalities	Tubal dysfunctions	Cervical dysfunctions
Anovulation	Amenorrhea	Frigidity
Stillbirth	Spontaneous abortion	

Why All The Stress?

Does stress lead to infertility, or does infertility cause stress, which then contributes to infertility? Psychology may not account for infertility in the early stages, but as a couple undergoes medical tests and all associated with trying to produce a baby on demand, the psychological may become a factor.

Some speculate that modernization is partly to blame for stress which interferes with the reproductive process. Researchers Gyongyossy and Szaloczy discovered that over a 20-year period in Hungary, the incidence of infertility cases related to anovulation increased from about 6 percent to 36 percent. They deduced that the increased stress was a result of modernization with its attendant fast-paced, high-pressure lifestyle.[82]

Another factor that can deepen stress for the infertile couple is the pressure applied by family members anxious for a grandchild, niece or nephew. Parents-in-law may think their child could have had children with another spouse. Your sense of frustration may heighten when you're around brothers and sisters with children.

Often family members say things without thinking. During one family get-together, an unmarried daughter told her father she never wanted to get married. In the presence of his infertile son and daughter-in-law he replied, "You have to get married! I want more grandchildren!" The daughter-in-law felt like she and her husband were a disappointment to his parents. One woman with severe financial limitations was told by a relative that she must not want kids as badly as someone willing to spend thousands of dollars on doctors and tests. Certainly no offense was intended by the comments, but when feelings are tender such comments only deepen the frustration and anxiety.

The most convincing evidence of the manner in which stress affects fertility is found during times of war. For example, it is not unusual for women to stop menstruating when their husbands go off to war. Many stop menstruating when subjected to the stress of bombing raids or concentration camps. While some such cases may be related to malnutrition during wartime, evidence exists that many cases are solely psychological in nature.

I've heard more than one story about women who conceived after they honestly stopped thinking about pregnancy. One woman had been trying to conceive for more than seven years. "I just got to the point I decided I wasn't going to worry about it, and then I got pregnant," she said.

Another woman had been trying for two years to get pregnant. "When I decided not to worry about it, I got pregnant," she reported. This same story is retold over and over. The clincher is, you can't force yourself to relax.

Robert M.L. Winston, Professor of Fertility Studies at the University of London cites cases of people who conceive soon after resolving deep emotional conflicts, going on vacations, quitting their jobs, and resolving other stressful situations.[83] Of course, quitting your job and going on a vacation may result in more stress in the long run if you neglect pressing responsibilities. However, if you can alleviate the stress in your life, your chances of conceiving might increase.

Fortunately, counseling or resolution of emotional problems often corrects stress-related infertility.

What Does Counseling Offer?

A story on the *CBS Evening News* reported that many infertile couples who undergo counseling succeed in conceiving, proving that for some couples, psychological factors can prevent conception.

A staff psychologist at the New England Deaconess Hospital in Boston, Alice Domar, has used relaxation techniques to overcome the tension and emotional pain associated with infertility. The technique Alice used was developed by a colleague, Herbert Benson, and is referred to as the "relaxation response." The method focuses on the physiological changes that accompany a relaxed mind.

Domar's patients participate in a 10-session program designed to incur deep relaxation through deep breathing, meditation and positive imagery. Women use the technique 20 minutes twice a day, always at the same time. Women are counseled to concentrate on a word or phrase that makes them feel better.

Domar hypothesizes that stress may worsen some infertility cases because of the body responses it triggers. For example, the hypothalamus, which regulates the flight or fight response, also regulates the ovaries through the pituitary gland. Some women, when under a great deal of stress, don't ovulate.

Speaking to *American Health* magazine, Domar cited a 1983 study in which 14 South American women with unexplained infertility underwent treatment. Seven received routine care, while seven underwent stress management and relaxation response therapy. After three months four of the women undergoing therapy were pregnant; none of the control patients were.[84]

For women interested in practicing relaxation therapy, the books "The Relaxation Response" and "Beyond the Relaxation Response" by Herbert Benson may prove very helpful.

Many other studies have documented a connection between counseling and increased fertility rates among couples with unexplained infertility. In her book, "Infertility: A Comprehensive Text," Machelle M. Seibel summarizes several studies which suggested that counseling helps many couples with unexplained infertility.

In one study, 16 patients had unexplained infertility and depression. They had been infertile from two to 11 years. Nine of the patients agreed to undergo therapy. Three of those who had experienced longstanding depression became pregnant. None of the patients who didn't receive counseling conceived.

In another study, women who had unexplained infertility for a minimum of three years met in group sessions for a period of four to six weeks. They discussed the subjects of marriage, sex, infertility tests, husbands, childlessness and other infertility issues. Many showed improved attitudes and sexual functioning. Twenty-one percent became pregnant within six months, and 26.5 percent became pregnant within the next several months.

Siebel cites another study in which five patients with unexplained infertility participated in a group discussion, sharing feelings of guilt, inadequacy and marital problems. Three of the five became pregnant.

Based on studies that followed the effects of counseling on unexplained infertility, 26.5 to 60 percent of couples become pregnant with counseling. Siebel summarized, "It appears that group therapy provides effective management for patients suffering from unexplained infertility; not only does it apparently provide major psychologic benefits, it may serve to increase the chance of conception."[85]

One researcher reported that about 35 percent of women having difficulty conceiving get pregnant soon after any form of psychological treatment is begun. In some cases the enthusiasm with which the woman is counseled is considered the therapeutic agent.[86]

Just Relax

I don't know how many people have told me those two most despicable words. At times I've thought the next person who told me to relax was going to get his or her lights punched out!

So how do you relax? One way is to accept your situation rather than fight it. This may sound like strange advice. Will accepting that you might never have children make the possibility of having them more likely? It might, if you can reach a state of calm acceptance. If you're constantly projecting hate thoughts toward your body for not working, you may create more problems than you need to have. This isn't my theory alone; I heard it from my doctor.

The question you need to answer is, are there emotional factors, even deep within you that you're barely aware of, that might create a block in your mind that may prevent you from having children?

Deep down, are you afraid of the responsibility children bring with them? Are you afraid you'll lose your freedom? Are you afraid you're not qualified to be a parent because of your own poor childhood? For women, do you harbor resentment toward your husband that might prevent you from "accepting" a child from him? It may sound far-fetched, but if emotional barriers are in your path, even subconsciously, they can affect your ability to conceive. Of course, no scientific test could ever prove this, but that doesn't mean it's not true.

A woman named Kathy told me she had been through almost all of the infertility diagnostic tests possible and her doctor was unable to find a reason for her infertility. (She easily conceived the first child, but tried for five years before the second one came along.) The person finally able to help her was, oddly enough, her chiropractor.

"He talked to me about feelings I had that might be keeping me from allowing myself to get pregnant. I found out that I harbored resentment toward my husband, and wouldn't completely 'give myself' to him. Those feelings interfered with my ability to conceive. The doctor wouldn't let me leave his office until I let go of those feelings."

As Kathy found out, chiropractors tend to have a holistic view of healing, and give more emphasis to the mind-body relationship than does the average physician. Kathy successfully conceived, for which she thanks her chiropractor.

Getting in Touch With Your Feelings

Many alternatives are open for the person who wants to explore whether psychological factors are interfering with conception, including therapists and naturopathic doctors.

A nationwide support group for infertile couples called RESOLVE can provide you with camaraderie and give you an outlet for your feelings. RESOLVE was founded in 1973 by Barbara Eck Menning. The organization serves as a counseling, referral and support system. Chapters are located in over 40 cities around the United States.

Check your local phone book for a RESOLVE chapter near you, or write:

> **RESOLVE, Inc.**
> **P.O. Box 474**
> **Belmont, MA 02178**
> **(617) 484-2424**

Some members of RESOLVE are former infertile couples who either conceived spontaneously or through therapy. The group support and opportunity to share your feelings with others in a similar situation may do you a world of good.

You may feel you need professional counseling. In the meantime, there are other outlets for your feelings of frustration.

Laughter Therapy?

"There ain't much fun in medicine, but there's a heck of a lot of medicine in fun." Those are the wise words of Josh Billings. And believe it or not, researchers have actually verified the medicinal value of laugter.

When we're feeling stressed, the body releases large doses of stress hormones. These hormones have a place—for example, when you need to run away from a rabid dog. But if you go about your daily life with high levels of stress hormones, the effects on your health (and your fertility) can be very detrimental. Studies show stress hormones supress the immune system and make us more vulnerable to disease.

Doctors Rod Martin and Herbert Lefcourt studied the connection between humor and the ability to adjust to major life stressors. Those with a good sense of humor were able to cope better with "tensions."[87] In another study at the Loma Linda University School of Medicine in California, male hospital workers were hooked up to catheters. Half the men watched a funny movie while the other half sat quietly in a room. Researchers collected blood samples every 10 minutes and analyzed them for immune-supressing hormones. They found that stress hormone levels remained constant in the control group but lowered in the group who watched the movie.

It's doubtful that laughter itself will cure infertility. However, filling your life with things that make you feel good and cultivating a healthy sense of humor may reduce your stress levels—and we've seen how stress can affect the reproductive system. Laughter seems to activate the release of endorphins, substances within the body which produce a feeling of well-being and stimulate the immune system.

The moral: Turn on those old "I Love Lucy" reruns or rent your favorite comedies and have a good chuckle. As one person put it, he who laughs, lasts.

Journal-Keeping

Another way to let out frustration is to write your feelings down. Journal-keeping has been recognized as one of the most effective therapies for all sorts of problems. Journal workshops are even conducted around the country for the purpose of helping people learn how to do their own psychological self-care. Many psychologists are incorporating journal-keeping in their patients' therapies. Some are calling it a breakthrough in mental health care.

Dr. Ira Progoff, who conducts journal workshops, said, "I see psychological self-reliance, or psychological self-care, a way of being able to tap into resources and knowledge within oneself that can enable us to deal with our problems, our experiences, in new ways. That's the principle I've tried to build into the Journal. . . I think people are much more capable of guiding their own efforts to get unstuck than we've given them credit for."[88]

Keeping a journal and evaluating your life's experiences can prove to be one of the most liberating therapies you've ever experienced. I'm not talking about simply keeping a daily diary with mundane events like those characterized in a "Leave it to Beaver" episode many years ago. Beaver's journal read something like this:

Monday

> Dear Diary: Got up. Ate breakfast. Went to school. Came home. Ate dinner. Went to bed.

Tuesday

> Dear Diary: Got up. Ate breakfast. Went to school. Came home. Ate supper. Went to bed.

You get the idea.

In order to experience the therapeutic benefits of journal writing, you must record your reactions to and feelings about events, not merely the events themselves. You don't necessarily need to write daily, or even about the present. You can explore your feelings about events that you experienced at any time in your life.

About two years ago I undertook the project of writing my life story. I had been feeling depressed and out of control, and wanted to come to terms with my life and see if I could make sense out of the events I was experiencing. Following the experts' advice, I wrote about isolated events—things like my favorite teacher, my most embarrassing moment, and so on—rather than trying to chronicle my life from the day I was born to the present.

I had experiences of overwhelming emotion as I wrote about my life's events stemming as far back as early childhood. The feelings and insights I gained from this writing experience helped me emerge from the rut of depression I'd been in for months. I saw my life with a new sense of purpose, and realized I could cope with infertility, as I had coped with other difficult experiences.

Try it! You might be surprised at the insights you'll gain. You may even be able to make sense of your experience with infertility.

For starters, buy a notebook or journal. Dr. Progoff, mentioned earlier, recommends that you begin by letting yourself relax for several minutes. Let your worries slip away. As your relaxation deepens, ask yourself "Where am I now in life?" Think about the present period of your life, whether it started with a new job, with your marriage, a move, or something else.

How do you feel about the current period of life you're in? You may feel like a dark cloud is hanging over your head, or like your hands are tied and you can't reach your goals. Don't judge or evaluate your thoughts, simply let them flow. Certain answers may enter your mind, such as when this period of your life started, and what events stand out. When you start to get some clear-cut feelings about this period of your life, perhaps some answers, start writing. Don't edit or criticize them—simply experience them.

Here are some questions you may want to answer with a paragraph or two:

1. When did you first suspect you were infertile? How did you feel?
2. Do you remember ever having any negative feelings about having children? Under what circumstances did you have these feelings?
3. Do you ever blame yourself for causing your infertility? Do you feel guilty about mistakes or sins in your past, and feel like you're being punished? What mistakes are they?
4. Express how you feel about being a mother or father. Write about your own childhood, and how you feel about your own parents.
5. Express any fears you might have about becoming a parent.
6. Before you started trying to have children, did you ever think you might not be able to conceive? Why?
7. Do you ever feel resentment toward your spouse that might make you "close yourself" off from him/her? What do you feel resentful about?
8. How did you feel about getting married? Were you scared, excited, nervous? Were you afraid of losing your independence?

Keeping a journal might prove to be the road to self-discovery you need to identify mental barriers you use to not allow yourself to become pregnant. Even if writing does not not help you to conceive, it can help you come to terms with the experience of infertility.

If you don't feel comfortable with the idea of paying to see a therapist, the closest thing to having your own psychologist is to keep a journal. Your inner voice can often offer you profound insights and wisdom no one else is capable of giving you.

For further help in journal self-therapy, obtain a copy of Dr. Progoff's book, "At a Journal Workshop."

Positive Ways to Handle Negative Emotions

Since it's been proven that emotions affect the reproductive cycle, what can you do to make sure your emotions don't work against you?

Obviously, deliberately trying not to think about getting pregnant is like trying not to think about breathing. Trying not to think about something keeps it foremost in your mind. But you can strive to develop a positive attitude and a calm response to the stressors that come your way. Here are a few ideas.

1. While lying in bed at night (or any other time you feel the need), picture a trash basket in the corner of the room until you have an image of one very clearly in your mind. Now visualize yourself getting out of bed (or your chair, etc), carrying your negative emotions in your arms, and walk over to the basket. Dump your worry, fear, anger, or other troublesome emotion into it. You can slam dunk it Michael Jordan style for more emphasis. Then turn around and leave your worries in the waste basket. Or, write your frustrations down on a piece of paper and throw it into the wastebasket. Or do like I did, and let your worries go up in smoke.

Early in my marriage I was troubled by the harsh reality of working full time, doing housework full time, being infertile, my occasional spats with my husband, the long road of school that lay ahead of him, financial frustrations and a host of other vague, unidentifiable problems that made me unhappy with life. I was unhappy with myself as well. In other words, the honeymoon was over!

One day my husband and I were out camping and he went on a hike by himself. I sat near the fire and for about two hours wrote down all the things that were troubling me. Then, looking at the fire, I decided to burn my worries away. I ripped up the papers (for extra emphasis) I had written and threw them in the fire. As I watched them burn away I felt the burden lift off my shoulders.

2. Keep a journal.

3. Write yourself a letter. Be completely honest about what you feel and how you want to feel. Give yourself a pep talk on paper.

4. Talk about your problems into a tape recorder, indulging yourself in self-pity if you desire. When you replay it, you might experience some interesting feelings. (I tried this one with another problem in my life. I

felt so silly listening to myself complain I didn't ever worry about that particular problem again.)

5. If you're angry or resentful with someone—perhaps your spouse, the pregnant woman you saw at the grocery store, or the "fertile Myrtle" in your family—write that person a letter, but destroy it when you're done. Often the very act of talking to the person on paper helps you to resolve your feelings. It's also a good release for the bottled-up anger.

6. Pray. "Come unto me, all ye that labor and are heavy laden, and I will give you rest," Jesus said (Matthew 11:28). Talk to God about your feelings, anger, challenges, or anything else. Talk to him as if he were there in the room with you.

7. Read the Bible or other inspirational literature. One of my all-time favorites is "The Power of Positive Thinking" by Norman Vincent Peale. Write down on note cards quotes or scriptures that make you feel happy and memorize them. Put them on your mirror, refrigerator or somewhere you'll see them every day.

8. Exercise. It's been scientifically proven that exercise releases substances called endorphins into the bloodstream, which give the exerciser an emotional lift.

9. Do something for someone else. To paraphrase Abe Lincoln, the best way to forget your own burdens is to relieve someone else's. Do volunteer service in the community. Give money or food to a homeless person. Visit an elderly folks' home. Read to the blind. Work for a crisis center. When you serve someone else, your own burden is lifted.

10. Count your blessings. It only takes a small dose of reality once in awhile to make me realize how fortunate I am. I'm not talking about a Pollyanna-type attitude that denies any pain or frustration in life, but rather a realistic acknowledgement of how good things are compared to how much worse they could be. Someone with a healthy sense of humor said, "Don't be disappointed when you don't get what you want; just be grateful you don't get what you deserve."

11. Don't blame life, God, family members, your spouse, or anyone else for your problems. The victim mentality, in my opinion, has done a great deal of damage to modern society. Take responsibility for making some-

thing out of your life. Helen Keller who, being blind and mute, had every reason to develop a victim mentality, said, "Keep your face to the sunshine and you cannot see the shadows."

12. Face a worst-case scenario and decide what your best self would do. Let's say you'll never have children. What will you do with your life? What do you want people to remember you for after your life is over? If you could do anything you want with your life (except for having children) what would you do? Of course, if you've planned your life and dreams around having a family, this exercise will be difficult. The fact is, nothing will substitute for a family. But if you never had one, would you want to look back and feel that you'd wasted your life in wishful thinking?

One day as I was planning a long-anticipated trip to the East Coast, I wondered what it would be like if I planned my daily life with the same enthusiasm. Life is like a long vacation—we're only here for a limited time. If we spend all our time criticizing what's wrong with the journey, we'll miss all the sights along the way.

The Healing Power of Faith and Prayer

Infertility—or barrenness—is a common theme in the Bible. Abraham, who was promised his seed would be as the sands of the seashore, was married to the barren Sarah. Imagine the faith it must have taken to believe God's promise to him would be fulfilled under such circumstances. When Sarah was told she would bear a child in her nineties, she laughed. She was chastised with the words, "Is anything too hard for the Lord?" (Genesis 18:14)

The theme of barrenness continues with many Bible heros and heroines such as Jacob and Rachel, Hanna in the book of Samuel, and Elisabeth in the New Testament. The poignant emotions these women experienced are captured in their stories and illustrate that God will not forget the barren. "He maketh the barren to keep house, and to be a joyful mother of children," the psalmist wrote (Psalm 113:9). He understands how you feel.

I would feel like I'd left something vital out of this book if I didn't put in a word for God. If you don't believe in God you can skip this section, but I hope you won't. If you're angry at God for not answering your prayers for a baby, don't skip this section. Because most people do believe in God, no book about health and personal problems would be complete without a discussion of the healing power of faith and prayer—and the miracles that can happen with God's help.

Thousands of couples who believe in God experience the pain of infertility, even after years of praying and pleading that He will send them a child. Others find that He miraculously answers their prayers for a child. Why does he answer some people in the affirmative, and not others? This may be one of the greatest challenges of faith a religious infertile couple could ever experience.

Like Abraham of the Old Testament, it seems each of us experiences profound trials of faith. Infertility may be yours, as it was Sarah's, Rachel's, Hannah's and Elizabeth's. Did God put these examples in the Holy Scriptures to comfort the barren? Surely He understands the depth of a woman's desire for children. Just knowing He understands can make the burden lighter.

I believe that in the long run, everything that happens is for our own benefit if we try to find the opportunities in our challenges. That optimism is not easy to feel in our darkest hours, but looking back we usually find it to be true. I would like to believe that everything I ask for God will grant me, but it doesn't happen that way. Sometimes things I want aren't in my best interest. And sometimes God makes our greatest trials turn out to be our greatest blessings.

Some couples have the distinct feeling God wants them to provide homes for children who need a chance, feeling that adoption is their unique mission in life. One infertile woman said, "A feeling of peace came over me one day after I felt the distinct impression that our mission in life was to adopt." Many, upon adopting, feel that the child was meant to be theirs, and observe a divine hand in the adoption process.

Infertile couples often examine their past misdeeds and sins, wondering if infertility is a punishment for things done wrong. I've come to realize that God is not punishing me by withholding children, but rather providing an opportunity if I'll look up and reach for it.

There's no healer like the great Healer, the one who created our bodies and the miracle of life. Asking God in faith for a child or a miraculous healing may bring you a miracle. Then again, the answer may be no. You may need to ask him not for physical healing, but for emotional healing. He does answer prayer—in His own way.

"Cast thy burden on the Lord, and he shall sustain thee." (Psalm 55:22)

Where Do You Go From Here?

Well, you've reached the end of the book, but you're at the beginning of your quest to take control of your own emotional and physical health. I hope you've enjoyed learning about nutrition and the mind-body connection. I hope you find the answers you're seeking. And I hope you'll continue to learn all you can about the things you can do to live a healthy, happy life.

I'm not anti-medicine or anti-doctor. Modern medicine has worked wonders in too many ways to count, and helped many people to conceive who otherwise wouldn't have been able to. But it is possible to combine the best of all worlds—doctors, nutrition, herbs, emotions and the spiritual dimension. Hopefully this book has added another dimension to your quest in overcoming infertility.

I would love to hear your success stories or comments on how this book can be improved. Please write to me at the publisher's address:

Karen Bradstreet
C/O Woodland Books
P.O. Box 1422
Provo, Utah 84603

Note: The information in these appendices is not purported to in any way overcome infertility, but rather to introduce you to the philosophy of natural health.

THE NATURAL HEALTH PHILOSOPHY: CLEANSING AND BUILDING

Simplistically speaking, the natural health philosophy is based on the idea that the human body is designed to protect and restore itself and will do so if it's not burdened with toxic overload. The philosophy also recognizes the important role the mind plays in health.

Years of poor dietary habits—including heavy consumption of refined grains, chemical additives, drugs and processed foods—can weaken the body's ability to cleanse and rebuild itself. With this type of diet the body is simply not getting the nutrients it needs to function optimally. Breakdown and disease occur.

When one's diet consists chiefly of refined and processed foods, the colon, the body's main organ of elimination, can become "polluted" and diseased. Without the dietary fiber necessary to aid the passage of and elimination of food through the body, pockets of old food, mucus and putrefaction can cling to the bowel walls. A state of autointoxication (self-poisoning) ensues. Natural health advocates believe autointoxication is the main reason for the high incidence of colon problems and degenerative diseases in the Western world.

When not properly eliminated from the body through the colon, toxins are absorbed back into the bloodstream and the body suffers from toxic overload. Fatigue, irritability, flatulence, nausea, constipation, irritable bowel, and more serious disease conditions can result as toxins that would normally be absorbed and eliminated through the colon remain in the body and cause degeneration.

Autopsies have revealed colons in grossly convoluted states, the result of a lifetime of poor eating habits. Many people, including myself, can attest to the benefits of a high-fiber diet rich in natural, unprocessed foods. Before ever experiencing female problems, I first experienced digestive problems. A doctor diagnosed me with spastic colon and gave me a medication to help my colon relax. I took one tablet and it made me so ill I didn't touch another one. Besides, I knew it didn't solve whatever was causing my problems.

I endured colon problems for three or four years until I learned about the natural health philosophy. With the simple addition of psyllium hulls (fiber) and food enzymes to my diet my digestive problems disappeared. I started to feel better than ever. As my intestinal health improved, my female problems began to disappear also.

In a nutshell, then, cleansing the colon is the basis for creating a more healthy state in the body. If you'd like to learn more about this aspect of health, natural food stores have many books on the subject. It is presented here simply as a sidelight. As I stated earlier, the autointoxication theory was commonly accepted before the advent of modern medicine.

Cleansing the colon will probably not directly solve your fertility problems, but it will help your body to rid itself of toxins that may have accumulated over the years. It will also help your body to absorb through the intestinal walls the nutrients it needs to function properly. It doesn't matter how well you eat if your body is unable to assimilate the nutrients or rid itself of toxins. Digestive enzymes can also be purchased which will help you assimilate the vitamins and minerals in your food.

Colon Cleansing

Many methods exist for cleansing the colon. The easier of these follow.

1.   This one is probably the easiest: Drink one teaspoon of psyllium hulls in juice three times daily. (Use a product without additives; the

most common brands contain sugar or aspartame. Check a reputable health food store.) Just this regimen alone continued over several weeks or months has the potential to remove deposits which have accumulated on the intestinal walls. Psyllium hulls swell several times their weight in water and cleanse the colon. They also absorb toxins for elimination. Scientists have found that regular use of psyllium hulls also lowers cholesterol.

You can continue using psyllium indefinitely. It is not habit-forming. My husband, who has met many natural health ideas with skepticism, is a loyal psyllium user.

2.   Supplementary herbs that help cleanse the colon:

Cascara sagrada (many over-the-counter laxatives contain this ingredient.)
Black walnut (helps eliminate parasites)
Pumpkin seeds (helps eliminate parasites)
Slippery elm (soothes inflammation; lubricates)

3.   Eat predominantly whole grains, fresh vegetables and fresh fruits. A few of my favorite healthy recipes are included in Appendix B. Learning how to eat healthy takes a little bit of effort, but once you reap the health benefits you'll be hooked.

General Cleanses

A cleanse is a temporary diet designed to help the body cleanse and detoxify itself. Instead of focusing its energies on digestion, during a cleanse the body is free to throw off toxins. Although often a person starting a cleanse will feel worse than normal at first, and experience symptoms such as nausea, headaches, colds, runny nose and so on, those who use cleanses attest to the wonderful, glowing way they feel after completing a cleanse.

Many in orthodox health fields mock those who claim going on a cleanse may make you sick at first as the body releases toxins into the bloodstream for elimination. These people will blame the herbs or the natural health philosophy for making you sick. I have to admit, I was skeptical until I went on a cleanse. I drank only fruit juices for several days and ate only natural foods. In addition, I drank a large volume of pure water. Like clockwork, I started to get symptoms of the flu and experienced tremendous mucus drainage—the likes of which I'd never before experienced in my life—for almost a week. I'd had annoying mucus in my throat for years and had been unable to get rid of it. After the initial flulike experience, I felt better than I had in years. Everything happened just like the naturalists predicted.

My personal favorite is the fruit juice/natural foods cleanse. I drink mostly fruit juices, but if I get hungry I can eat fresh fruits or vegetables, baked potatoes or brown rice.

Here are a few mild cleanses to help your body throw out toxins which may have accumulated during years of poor eating habits. If you stick with it, you'll feel better than ever!

Fruit Juice Cleanse

Drink only fruit juices for anywhere from a day to a week. Fresh juices directly from the fruit are best; frozen are least desirable but they will still offer benefits if they're all you can come by. If you follow the juice cleanse for only a day, you won't reap quite the cleansing benefits you would from a more prolonged juice cleanse. You can drink fresh-squeezed lemon juice in water for additional cleansing.

Lemon Water-Cayenne Pepper-Maple Syrup Cleanse

My mother-in-law swears by this cleanse, and her children think it's one of the reasons she's been so healthy all of her life. She says she never feels better than when on the cleanse. It is somewhat more difficult to stick with than other cleanses, but if you can you'll feel all the better.

She didn't know where it came from, but I later discovered it has been attributed to Stanley Burroughs and is called the Master Cleanser.

2 T. fresh lemon or lime juice (not bottled)
2 T. pure maple syrup (Grade D best)
1/10 t. cayenne pepper
10 ounces hot or cold pure water

Mix all ingredients. Drink 6 to 12 glasses daily. Do not eat or drink anything else. Ideally, this cleanse should be continued for 10 days.

Natural Foods Diet

This is milder and easier to follow. Eat nothing but fresh fruits, vegetables, and whole grains for several weeks. You can eat whatever and as much as you want. Your body willl love you for it, and you'll feel more energetic than ever! Example: Eat a smoothie for breakfast, brown rice with veggies for lunch, and a salad for dinner.

Seven Days Miracle Diet

Someone gave this to me several years ago, and swore by it.

Day 1: Eat all fruits except bananas, as much as you want. Canteloupe and watermelon are especially good.

Day 2: All vegetables, raw uncooked. Green leafy vegetables are best. You may also have one baked potato with real butter.

Day 3: Fruits and vegetables, as much as you want. No potato.

Day 4: Bananas and skim milk. Eat as many as eight bananas and six glasses of skim milk. Also, as much T-J soup (below) as desired.

Day 5: Beef and tomatoes. Eat 10 - 12 ounces cooked beef and six tomatoes. Try to drink eight glasses of water.

Day 6: Beef and vegetables — as much as desired.

Day 7: Brown rice and unsweetened fruit juice and vegetables.

T-J Soup:

6 onions	1 can tomatoes
2 green peppers	1 head cabbage
1 stalk celery	

Cut into pieces, and simmer until vegetables are soft. Season with herbs.

You can develop healthy eating habits gradually—and although many nutritional purists would argue, common sense says ice cream or french fries now and then won't hurt you if the bulk of your diet is healthy.

Simple substitutions often go a long way. Start by buying more fresh produce, and eat more vegetables. Eat fruits and whole grains for breakfast. Use whole wheat bread instead of white bread; buy unbleached and whole wheat flour instead of white flour. Use brown rice instead of white rice. Use more beans, lentils and other legumes. Eat more stir-fried vegetables and Oriental meals. Make vegetable-based soups more often. Snack on vegetables and fruits, including dried fruits, more often than cookies and potato chips.

One thing that always amazed me when I lived in France was how slender and long-lived the French were, yet they ate plenty of buttery sauces and plenty of food in general. They didn't seem at all preoccupied with cholesterol, fat, sugar, and other American panic buttons. They eat cheese like it's going out of style (there's a variety for every day of the year), a great deal of yogurt and lots of egg dishes. Their incidence of heart disease is so low that they were featured on a special CBS *60 Minutes* story.

I'm not saying the French are the healthiest or most fertile people in the world, but they do seem to enjoy longevity and lack of weight problems. Perhaps best of all, they have a healthy attitude toward food. There were several key things I noticed about French eating habits as compared to American eating habits:

1. They snack very little between meals as compared to Americans, who plop down in front of the TV armed with potato chips, cookies, soda pop and beer.
2. They take a long time to eat their meals and thoroughly enjoy eating.
3. They eat fresh vegetables abundantly.
4. They eat very few processed foods. Many go to the market daily to

buy fresh foods which are prepared the same evening. I think this especially is a key to good health—fresh, unprocessed foods. Americans have largely gotten away from wholesome, fresh meals cooked from scratch.

5. Their pastries are not nearly as sweet as are ours, nor do the French consume nearly as much sugar. Most desserts are fruit-based.

6. They drink a great deal of mineral water (such as Perrier) and very little tap water.

7. They eat an enormous variety of foods. (They eat for salads anything that's green. Add a little vinaigrette [see recipe below] and it becomes a gourmet dish.)

8. They have a rich tradition of herbal use and natural health care is widely accepted. Herbal remedies sit alongside modern medical remedies in pharmacies.

If we desire optimal health, we can learn from the French way of eating. The Oriental way of eating, of course, has also been recognized as one of the healthiest cuisines, with its emphasis on vegetables and practice of eating meat in moderation.

A FEW HEALTHY RECIPES

Brown Rice and Steamed Vegetables for Two

1. Cook 1 cup raw brown rice according to package directions. You may add some chicken bouillon for flavor.

2. For 15 minutes steam, in a large pot, coarsely cut up carrots, broccoli, cauliflower, onions, and anything else you desire.

3. Saute 2 c. mushrooms in 1-2 tablespoons real butter with two or three minced garlic cloves and three or four shakes soy sauce.

Serve steamed vegetables over rice and smother with mushrooms. You may sprinkle with grated cheddar cheese if desired, and season with soy sauce.

Variation: Serve steamed vegetables and sauted mushrooms on baked potatoes. Sprinkle with grated cheddar cheese.

Pinto Beans and Rice

Soak 2 c. pinto beans (or any beans, for that matter) overnight and cook the next day according to directions with the ingredients that follow. Chop one whole onion, three or four garlic cloves, 2 stalks celery, two carrots and add to beans while cooking. Season with Season All or vegetable seasoning to taste. Add a large slab of turkey ham or use stock flavoring while cooking. When beans are almost done, remove the slab of turkey ham and add about one cup bite-sized pieces of turkey ham. Serve over brown rice.

Variation: Use lentils instead of beans.

Couscous

Boil one chicken, skin removed, in about eight cups water with 1 chopped onion and 2 minced garlic cloves. When done, remove the meat from the bones and set aside. Reserve broth. To the broth add 2 carrots cut in 1-inch chunks, 1/2 head cauliflower cut in florettes, 1 can garbanzo beans (chick peas), 1 zucchini cut in 1/2 inch slices, 2-3 fresh tomatoes cut in chunks, chunked turnips (optional), and chicken meat. Season to taste with Season All, 1/2 teaspoon cayenne pepper, salt and 1/2 teaspoon chili powder (broth should have a little "bite"). Boil until vegetables are tender. Correct the seasoning. Prepare 1 box couscous according to package directions. Spoon stew mixture over couscous and enjoy.

Smoothies
(Great for breakfast, lunch or dinner)

Recipe for one person

Put in a blender one ripe banana, broken into three or four chunks.
To the banana add any two of the following:

1 washed peach, cut into four chunks, seed removed
5 washed strawberries with tops removed
One peeled orange
1/4 c. pitted cherries

Add 8 oz. fruit juice of your choice, 1-2 cups ice, and blend until completely smooth. You may add 1/4 to 1/2 cup plain yogurt, wheat bran, or anything your imagination allows. Enjoy!

Raw Spinach Salad

At least 1/2 hour ahead of time make the following vinaigrette:

3 T. vegetable oil (natural cold pressed or olive best)
1 T. cider vinegar
1-2 cloves minced garlic
1 teaspoon salt
Dash Pepper

Shake well and leave at room temperature for flavors to mix.

Wash enough raw spinach to make a salad the size of your choice. Dry and tear gently into a bowl. Shake vinaigrette and correct the seasoning. If necessary, add salt or more vinegar. When seasoning is correct shake well and pour over spinach. Toss well. You may not need all of the vinaigrette; don't overdo it. Sprinkle generously with Parmesan cheese and mix. Add 1-2 c. croutons (garlic-onion flavor is delicious) and toss lightly. Eat immediately; spinach will wilt within several minutes.

Note: This vinaigrette is delicious on virtually any kind of salad, including pasta salad made with plenty of fresh vegetables.

Tomato-Cucumber Salad

Make vinaigrette, above. Thinly slice two or three tomatoes and a cucumber. Pour some of the vinaigrette on a serving platter and arrange cucumbers and tomatoes in an attractive pattern. Cover with remaining vinaigrette. Slice in half three boiled eggs and arrange on top of tomato slices. Garnish eggs with a dab of mayonnaise and paprika. Garnish platter with parsley, if desired. Yummy!

Avocado & Sprouts on Whole Wheat Bread

Toast two pieces of whole wheat bread. Spread one slice with mayonnaise. Halve an avocado and remove the seed and skin. Cut in thin slices and arrange on one of the pieces of toasted bread. Sprinkle with garlic salt or a pinch of cayenne pepper if desired. Top with a hearty amount of alfalfa sprouts and the other piece of toasted bread. Delicious!

Green Drinks

In a blender, combine 12 ounces pineapple juice with any kind of washed greens—carrot tops, spinach, alfalfa sprouts, and herbs if desired. Blend and drink. The green drink takes some getting used to, but you'll love the way you feel after drinking one. Nothing could be healthier for you—and if you get pregnant, for your baby.

(One time I made the mistake of combining freshly picked alfalfa, banana, carrots and apple juice. Although it made me feel energetic almost instantly after drinking it, the combination looked and tasted terrible! Whatever you do, don't add a banana!)

Appendix C

FASTING

"Instead of using medicine, fast." *Aesculapius, ancient Greek philosopher*

Fasting has been used for both religious and health purposes for centuries. Fasting's health benefits are the main concern here, although I can attest to the spiritual benefits of fasting as well. Fasting can clear the mind, create a feeling of well-being, and sharpen the intellect. When I have a problem that seems to be getting the best of me, fasting never fails to help me gain a new strength and perspective.

But what about fasting's physical benefits? Given the chance, the body is able to throw off dangerous toxins. By instinct the body rejects food when very sick to give itself a chance to focus its energies on fighting off whatever is making it sick. Even animals, when sick, will not eat, or they will instinctively eat certain plants (such as cats eating grass). When the body's energies aren't focused on digestion, they can be directed toward house-cleaning.

Fasting is defined differently in many different circles. Among some, fasting is completely abstaining from food or drink. Among others, fasting is partaking only of liquid. Among still others, fasting is eating only lightly, or eating only after sundown. For our purposes here, fasting is the elimination of solid food from the diet.

What to Expect During a Fast

The cleansing process begins when you miss the first meal, and usually reaches its maximum effects on the third day. However, even 24-hour fasts will give your body a rest and allow some house-cleaning to take place.

Because during the fast the body is throwing off toxins into the bloodstream, many people experience bad breath, headaches, muscular aches, a coated tongue and flulike symptoms. The sooner you feel poorly, the more toxins you've accumulated in the body. Some people cannot miss even one meal without experiencing a headache. People in this category are most in need of fasting.

When the symptoms subside you'll experience a clarity of mind and feeling of well-being that makes fasting very gratifying.

When you fast for more than three days, you will usually enter a deeper cleanse after the period of well-being, in which the body is throwing off toxins at an even deeper level. You may feel tired, have difficulty thinking and feel muscle aches or other symptoms. Once these pass you'll again experience a wonderful sense of health, vitality and well-being.

TYPES OF FASTS

Several sample fasts are included here. Check with your health expert before undergoing fasts of more than three days. Because each individual is different, fasting is a very personal issue. What is right for another may not be right for you. Some people easily tolerate prolonged fasts, while others in a weakened condition can barely tolerate a day's fast.

A note about breaking fasts: If you break your fast with a huge, rich dinner, you'll lose many of the benefits of fasting. Ease into regular eating habits. It is best to break a fast with juices and natural foods such as steamed vegetables for a day or two.

24-Hour Fast

• Abstain from any type of food or drink for 24 hours. When you break the fast, eat lightly and only natural foods, especially fruit or vegetables. Ease into a normal meal schedule.

Water Fast

I have a friend whose mother occasionally went on seven-day water fasts, and claimed she never felt better than when on the fast.

• Drink only purified water for one to seven days. You must be in proper condition for this fast. It is definitely not recommended for those in weak health.

Fruit Juice Fast

On a juice fast, you can choose to drink only one type of juice or many types.
• Drink only fruit juice from one to seven days.
• Drink only fresh lemon juice squeezed in water from one to seven days.

Vegetable Juice Fast

• Drink only vegetable juice from one to seven days.

Many books dedicated exclusively to fasting are available in health food stores and libraries. This section is intended to be an introduction rather than an in-depth discussion. Visit your library or bookstore for more information.

RISKS OF DRUGS COMMONLY USED TO TREAT INFERTILITY

(information from the 1992 Physician's Desk Reference)

Bromocriptine

Used to treat: amenorrhea, galactorrhea, elevated prolactin
Potential side effects: nausea, headache, vomiting, fatigue, dizziness, light-headedness, nasal congestion, constipation, diarrhea, drowsiness; fainting, seizures, stroke, low blood pressure, shortness of breath, hallucinations, disturbed dreams.
Trade name: Parlodel

Danocrine (danazol)

Used to treat: endometriosis, fibrocystic breast disease
Potential side effects: weight gain, acne, seborrhea, hirsutism (excess hair growth in unusual places), water retention, hair loss, voice change, spotting, amenorrhea, flushing, vaginal dryness, reduction in breast size, nervousness, emotional swings, jaundice, headache, dizziness, cataracts, pelvic pain, visual disturbances, masculinizing effects, birth defects and many others.

Synarel (nasal spray)

Used to treat: endometriosis
Potential side-effects: ovarian cysts, abnormal vaginal bleeding, birth defects, hot flashes, emotional disturbances, decreased sex-drive, vaginal dryness, acne, reduction in breast size, irreversible loss in bone density, nasal irritation.

Note: This drug has never been tested for safety beyond six months of use.

Metrodin (injected)

Used to treat: stimulates follicular growth; must be combined with human chorionic gonadotropin to induce ovulation.

Potential side effects: abnormal ovarian enlargement; overstimulation of the ovary leading to life-threatening complications such as accumulation of fluid in the peritoneal cavity, thorax and pericardium, respiratory distress, pulmonary embolism, stroke, multiple births, headache, gastrointestinal upset, breast tenderness, hair loss, skin problems, birth defects, ectopic pregnancy, permanent damage to ovaries, has caused in death in some cases.

Pergonal

Used to treat: stimulates follicular growth; must be combined with human chorionic gonadotropin to induce ovulation.

Potential side-effects: abnormal ovarian enlargement; overstimulation of the ovary leading to life-threatening complications such as accumulation of fluid in the peritoneal cavity, thorax and pericardium, respiratory distress, pulmonary embolism, stroke, multiple births, headache, gastrointestinal upset, breast tenderness, hair loss, skin problems, birth defects, ectopic pregnancy, permanent damage to ovaries.

Profasi

Used to treat: induces ovulation in women who have been treated with Pergonal.

Potential side-effects: overstimulation of the ovary, sudden ovarian enlargement, rupture of ovarian cysts with effusion of blood into the peritoneal cavity, multiple births, blockage in the arteries, fluid retention, irritability, headache, restlessness, depression, fatigue, water retention, pain at the site of injection.

Serophene (Clomiphene)

Used to treat: induces ovulation in women with indications of normal estrogen production.

Potential side-effects: visual disturbances, multiple births, birth defects, overstimulation of the ovaries with attendant risks, hot flushes, abdominal discomfort, breast tenderness, nausea, vomiting, nervousness, insomnia, ovarian cyst formation, dizziness, depression, fatigue, abnormal uterine bleeding, weight gain, hair loss.

Birth-Control Pills

Used to treat: endometriosis

Potential side-effects: blood clots, heart attacks, rupture of blood vessels in the brain, cerebral thrombosis, hypertension, gallbladder disease, liver tumors, nausea, vomiting, abdominal cramps, bloating, breakthrough bleeding, spotting, amenorrhea, change in menstrual flow, temporary infertility after discontinuance, water retention, discoloration of the skin, breast changes, weight loss or increase, change in cervical erosion and secretion, loss of milk when given immediately after birth, jaundice, migraine, rash, depression, reduced tolerance of carbohydrates, Candida infection, change in cornea of the eye, intolerance to contact lenses, premenstrual syndrome, cataracts, appetite changes, headache, cystitislike symptoms, nervousness, dizziness, abnormal hair growth, loss of scalp hair, acne, colitis, others.

adhesions, endometrial growths in areas other than the uterus such as on ovaries and fallopian tubes, which can cause pain and damage reproductive organs.

amenorrhea, the absence of menstrual flow.

anovulation, lack of production of and discharge of an ovum by the ovary.

artificial insemination, mechanical injection of seminal fluid within the vagina or cervix.

azoospermia, absence of sperm in the semen.

bromocriptine, a drug often prescribed to suppress prolactin production and restore ovulation and menstruation in infertile women.

Candida albicans, a yeast fungus which normally resides in the intestinal and genitourinary tracts and on the skin.

cervical mucus, mucus produced around the time of ovulation designed to aid the passage of sperm and enhance the chances of fertilization; it may malfunction and hinder fertilization.

Chlamydia, a group of sexually transmittable microorganisms that often cause infertility and sometimes permanent sterility.

chocolate cysts, endometrial cysts located on the ovary which are filled with a fluid the consistency of chocolate syrup.

cilia, hairlike projections that help in the transport of the egg.

clomiphene, a non-steroidal drug used to stimulate ovulation.

clumping, grouping of sperm, negatively affecting their ability to move.

corpus luteum, a small yellow body that develops within a ruptured ovarian follicle. It secretes progesterone.

danazol, a drug often prescribed for the management of endometriosis which acts at least in part by inhibiting estrogen production.

DES (diethylstilbestrol), a synthetic drug several times more potent than natural estrogens used in the treatment of menopause and estrogen-related disorders. Has been found to cause vaginal problems and infertility in daughters whose mothers took the drug during pregnancy.

dyspareunia, pain during sexual intercourse.

dysmenorrhea, painful menstruation; experienced by about 50 percent of menstruating women. May be due to structural problems or hormone imbalances.

endocrine glands, any gland such as the thyroid or pituitary gland which secretes hormones into the blood or lymph.

endometriosis, the presence of uterine lining in other locations in the body, especially the ovaries, fallopian tubes and other pelvic organs; characterized by cyst formations and adhesions, and often causing severe pain.

epididymis, a small oblong structure which rests upon and behind the posterior section of the testes.

estrogen, a female hormone produced primarily by the ovaries; initiates the menstrual cycle, produces female secondary sex characteristics, and prepares the uterus for a fertilized egg.

fast, for the purposes of this book, abstinence from food for a specific period of time for the purpose of allowing the body to cleanse itself of toxins and allowing the healing mechanism to function more efficiently.

first-degree infertility, the inability to conceive or bear a child by an individual or couple who has never had children.

follicle stimulating hormone (FSH), a hormone produced by the anterior pituitary gland that stimulates the development of Graafian follicles in females and sperm in males.

galactorrhea, flow of milk after cessation of nursing or by a woman who has not had a baby.

galactorrhea-amenorrhea syndrome, breast secretion and absence of menstruation in a woman who is not pregnant or nursing.

goiter, an enlargement of the thyroid gland on the front and sides of the neck; indicative of low thyroid function.

growth hormones, artificial hormones given to animals to make them grow faster and bigger, produce more milk, etc. Their safety to humans who consume animal products has not been adequately confirmed.

hirsutism, excessive hair growth in unusual places, especially in women.

hyperprolactinemia, excessive secretion of prolactin often causing infertility, amenorrhea and galactorrhea.

hypothyroidism, condition produced by a deficiency in thyroid secretion by the thyroid gland.

impotence, the inability to maintain or sustain an erection.

in-vitro fertilization, the technique by which an ovum is fertilized with a sperm in a laboratory and implanted in a uterus for gestation.

luteal phase defect, lack of sufficient progesterone to maintain a pregancy in the second half of the menstrual cycle.

lutenizing hormone (LH), a hormone produced by the pituitary that acts upon the ovary to stimulate the ripening of a follicle and formation of the corpus luteum.

Mittelschmertz, pain felt at the site of the ovary during ovulation.

motility, the ability of sperm to swim; often calculated in sperm tests.

natural health, the philosophy that the body's healing mechanisms function most effectively through holistic measures such as proper nutrition and a healthy mental attitude.

oligospermia, deficient amount of sperm in seminal fluid necessary for fertilization; may be temporary or permanent.

oogenesis, formation and development of the ovum.

ovarian follicle, a small ovarian sac containing a maturing ovum.

ovum, the female reproductive cell, ie., egg.

pelvic inflammatory disease (PID), an inflammation of the female pelvic organs, usually the fallopian tubes, usually caused by bacteria.

post-coital test, test which samples the cervial mucus after intercourse to determine whether there are enough viable sperm present to fertilize an egg.

progesterone, a female hormone manufactured mostly by the ovaries that prepares the lining of the uterus for a fertilized ovum.

prolactin, a pituitary hormone that stimulates milk production.

prostaglandins, unsaturated fatty acids that play a role in the contraction of smooth muscle, the regulation of body temperature, the control of inflammation and many other functions.

secondary infertility, the inability to conceive or carry a pregnancy to term by one who has previously had a child or children.

T-mycoplasma, a tiny bacteria that lives in colonies in the urogenital tract; can cause infertility.

testosterone, a hormone secreted by the testes that stimulates the development of male sex organs, secondary sex characteristics and sperm production.

urethra, a duct that conveys urine from the bladder and also conveys semen.

variocele, a varicose vein in the scrotum that negatively affects sperm production.

vas deferens, a duct that transports sperm from the epididymus to the penis.

Bibliography

Barnes, Broda O. *Hypothyroidism: The Unsuspected Illness*, New York, NY: Harper & Row Publishers, 1976.

Bricklin, Mark. *The Practical Encyclopedia of Natural Healing*, Emmaus, PA: Rodale Press, 1983.

Corson, Stephen L. *Conquering Infertility*, East Norwalk, CT: Appleton-Century-Crofts, 1983.

Doctor's Book of Home Remedies. Deborah Tkac, Ed., Emmaus, PA: Rodale Press, 1990.

Fenton, Judith Alsofrom. *The Fertility Handbook*, New York, NY: Clarkson N. Potter, Inc., 1980.

Griffith, Winter H. *Complete Guide to Vitamins, Minerals & Supplements*, Tucson AZ: Fisher Books, 1988.

Heinerman, John. *Science of Herbal Medicine*, Orem, UT: Bi-World Publishers, 1984.

McFalls, Joseph A. *Psychopathology and Subfecundity*, New York, NY: Academic Press, 1979.

Medical Self-Care: Access to Health Tools. Tom Ferguson, Ed., New York: Summit Books, 1980.

Michaud, Ellen and Anastas, Lila L. *Listen to Your Body*, Emmaus, PA: Rodale Press, 1988.

Mills, Simon Y. *The Dictionary of Modern Herbalism,* Rochester, VT: Healing Arts Press, 1988.

Mindell, Earl. *Unsafe at any Meal,* New York, NY: Warner Books, 1987.

New Illustrated Medical Encyclopedia and Guide to Family Health, Robert E. Rothenberg, Ed., Danbury, CT: Grolier, Incorporated, 1988.

Ojeda, Linda. *Exclusively Female: A Nutrition Guide for Better Menstrual Health,* Claremont, CA: Hunter House Publishers, 1983.

Quillin, Patrick. *Healing Nutrients,* Chicago, IL: Contemporary Books, 1987.

Reproductive Toxicology. R.L. Dixon, Ed., New York, NY: Raven Press, 1985.

Rochlitz, Steven. *Allergies and Candida with the Physicist's Rapid Solutions,* New York, NY: Human Ecology Balancing Science, Inc., 1991.

Salaman, Maureen. *Foods that Heal.* Manlo Park, CA: Statford Publishing, 1989.

Sex, Birth & Babies. George Constable, Ed., Chicago, IL: Time Life Books, 1982.

Siebel, Machelle M. *Infertility: A Comprehensive Text,* East Norwalk, CT: Appleton & Lange, 1990.

Stangel, John. *The New Fertility and Conception: The Essential Book for Childless Couples,* New York, N.Y., New American Library, 1988.

Tenney, Louise. *Nutritional Guide with Food Combining.* Provo, UT: Woodland Books, 1991.

Tenney, Louise. *Today's Herbal Health,* Provo, UT: Woodland Books, 1983.

Thomas, Eric and Rock, John. *Modern Approaches to Endometriosis,* Lancaster, UK: Kluwer Academic Publishers, 1991.

Trattler, Ross. *Better Health Through Natural Healing: How to Get Well Without Drugs or Surgery,* McGraw-Hill Book Company, 1985.

Wade, Carlson. *The Natural Way to Health Through Controlled Fasting,* New York, NY: Arco Publishing Co., 1968.

Winston, Robert M.L. *What We Know About Infertility: Diagnosis, Treatment and Alternatives,* New York, NY: The Free Press, 1987.

Winter, Ruth. *A Consumer's Dictionary of Food Additives,* New York: Crown Publishers, Inc., 1978.

Wright, Jonathan V. *Dr. Wright's Book of Nutritional Therapy,* Emmaus, PA: Rodale Press, Emmaus, 1979.

Wright, Jonathan V. *Dr. Wright's Guide to Healing with Nutrition,* Emmaus, PA: Rodale Press, 1984.

Footnotes

[1]"Infertility Test Scores Low," *American Journal of Obstetrics & Gynecology,* 162:3, 615-20.

[2]Machelle M. Siebel, *Infertility: A Comprehensive Text* (East Norwalk, CT:Appleton & Lange, 1990), 7-9.

[3]Dean Black, Ph.D., "Candida: Our Unruly Guest," *The Healing Currents Series* (Springville, UT: Tapestry Press, 1989) 1.

[4]John Parks Trowbridge and Morton Walker, *The Yeast Syndrome,* (New York, NY: Bantam Books, 1986) 115.

[5]Ibid., 115.

[6]Dennis Remington and Barbara Higa, *Back to Health: A Comprehensive Medical and Nutritional Yeast Control Program* (Provo, UT: Vitality House International, Inc, 1991)216.

[7]John Parks Trowbridge and Morton Walker, *The Yeast Syndrome,* (New York, NY: Bantam Books, 1986) 330-331.

[8]Dean Black, Ph.D., "Candida, Our Unruly Guest," The Healing Currents Series (Springville, UT: Tapestry Press, 1989) 5.

[9]Dennis Remington and Barbara Higa, *Back to Health: A Comprehensive Medical and Nutritional Yeast Control Program* (Provo, UT: Vitality House International, Inc, 1991)216.

[10]Broda O. Barnes and Lawrence Galton, *Hypothyroidism: The Unsuspected Illness* (New York, NY: Harper & Row, Publishers, 1976) 135.

[11]Ibid.

[12]James F. Scheer, "Multiplying Chances for Conception: Sensible Solutions for Infertility Problems," *Health Freedom News,* January, 1992, 10.

[13]"A Cure for Infertility," *Chimo,* February, 1981, 59.

[14]Ellen Michaud and Lila L. Anastas, *Listen to Your Body* (Emmaus, PA: Rodale Press, Inc., 1988), 333.

[15]*The Deseret News,* Salt Lake City, Utah, Thursday, PM/Friday AM, March 3-4, 1983.

[16]Louise Tenney, *Louise Tenney's Nutritional Guide with Food Combining* (Provo, UT: Woodland Books, 1991), 132.

[17]"Danazol as a Treatment of Endometriosis," in *Modern Approaches to Endometriosis*, Edited by Eric Thomas and John Rock (Lancaster, UK: Kluwer Academic Publishers, 1991) 250.

[18]"Endometriosis and Infertility," in *Modern Approaches to Endometriosis*, Edited by Eric Thomas and John Rock (Lancaster, UK: Kluwer Academic Publishers, 1991) 121-122.

[19]Michael Kilpatrick, "Infertility was Our Problem," *Prevention*, April, 1981, 91-93.

[20]Maureen Salaman, *Foods that Heal* (Menlo Park, CA: Statford Publishing, 1989),330.

[21]Ibid., 329.

[22]John A. McDougall, "The 80% Solution," *Vegetarian Times*, May, 1990, 18.

[23]Journal of Urology, 137:1168, 1987.

[24]"Pyridoxine for Impotency?" *Better Nutrition*, August, 1979, 8-9.

[25]Robert E. Rothenberg, M.D., Ed., *The New Illustrated Medical Encyclopedia and Guide to Family Health* (Danbury, CT: Grolier, Inc., 1988), 1190-1196.

[26]John A Myers, "Minerals for Fertility," *Let's Live*, October, 1980, 26-38.

[27]Ralph B. Gwatkin, "Effects of Chemicals on Fertilization," in *Reproductive Toxicology*, R.L. Dixon, Ed. (New York, NY: Raven Press, 1985) 215.

[28]John Yates, "A Diet for Improved Sexuality," *Prevention*, December, 1979, 65-70.

[29]Emil Steinberger and James A. Lloyd, "Chemicals Affecting the Development of Reproductive Capacity," in *Reproductive Toxicology*, R.L. Dixon, Ed. (New York, NY: Raven Press, 1985), 2.

[30]Eileen Mazer, "Weak Seed," *Prevention*, June, 1980, 103.

[31]Machelle M. Siebel, *Infertility: A Comprehensive Text* (East Norwalk, CT: Appleton & Lange, 1990), 14.

[32]Lancet, no. 8626, 1453. Reported in "Caffeine Contraception," *East West,* June, 1989, 11.

[33]Betty Kamen, "Nutrition Dialogue," *Let's Live,* November, 1982, 96-97.

[34]Susan D. Schrag and Robert L. Dixon, "Reproductive Effects of Chemical Agents," in *Reproductive Toxicology,* R.L. Dixon, Ed. (New York, NY: Raven Press, 1985), 302.

[35]Eileen Mazer, "Weak Seed," *Prevention,* June, 1980, 103.

[36]Adelle Davis, *Let's Get Well* (New York NY: Harcourt, Brace & World, Inc., 1965), 212.

[37]"Links Flame Retardant, Fertility," *Health Fact News,* February, 1981, 4.

[38]Susan D. Schrag and Robert L. Dixon, "Reproductive Effects of Chemical Agents," in *Reproductive Toxicology,* R.L. Dixon, Ed. (New York, NY: Raven Press, 1985), 308-310.

[39]Ruth Winter, *A Consumer's Dictionary of Food Additives,* (New York, NY: Crown Publishers, Inc., 1978).

[40]*The Wellness Encyclopedia,* (Boston, MA: Houghton Mifflin Co, 1991), 184.

[41]*Medical Aspects of Human Sexuality,* Volume 13:10, October, 1979, 134.

[42]Carolyn Reuben and Joan Priestly, "Vitamins Against Miscarriage," *East West Magazine,* January, 1989, 59-62.

[43]Jonathan Wright, M.D., *Dr. Wright's Book of Nutritional Therapy* (Emmaus, PA: Rodale Press, Inc., 1979), 10.

[44]Journal of Clinical Endocrinology and Metabolism, June, 1976. Reported in John Yates' "A Diet for Improved Sexuality," *Prevention,* December, 1979, 65.

[45]Mark Bricklin, *The Practical Encyclopedia of Natural Healing* (Emmaus, PA: Rodale Press, Inc., 1983) 303-304.

[46]*The Vitamin E Fact Book,* Vitamin E Research and Information Service, 1989, 20.

[47]Robert Vare, "All About Vitamin E," 140. (Source of article not obtainable.)

[48]John Christopher, *Dr. Christopher's Newsletter,* 1979, 6. (Month not given.)

[49]John Yates, "A Diet for Improved Sexuality," Prevention, December, 1979, 65-69.

[50]Patrick Quillin, *Healing Nutrients* (Chicago, IL: Contemporary Books, 1987), 274.

[51]"Vitamin C Reverses Infertility," *Today's Living,* September, 1983, 13-14, 48-50.

[52]International Journal of Fertility, Vol. 22, no. 3, 1977.

[53]Carolyn Reuben and Joan Priestly, "Vitamins Against Miscarriage," *East West Magazine,* January, 1989, 61.

[54]Family Practice News, March 15, 1974. Reported in John Yates', "Bioflavonoids—They're Here to Make Us Healthier," *Prevention,* June, 1979, 138.

[55]Stephen Langer, M.D., "Vitamin A Influences Thyroid Function," *Better Nutrition,* December 1989, 14-15.

[56]Biology of Reproduction, November, 1979. Reported in Eileen Mazer's "Weak Seed," *Prevention,* June, 1980,103.

[57]James F. Scheer, "Selenium: The Mineral Marvel," *Health Freedom News,* March, 1991, 26-27.

[58]"The Physiochemical Role of Chelated Minerals," *Journal of Applied Nutrition,* 16-17.

[59]Herbert H. Boynton, "Selenium: Powerful New Weapon Against Disease," *The American Chiropractor,* January, 1979, 52-53.

[60]Uhland A., Kwiecinski G., DeLuca H., "Normalization of Serum Calcium Restores Fertility in Vitamin D-Deficient Male Rats," *Journal of Nutrition,* 122:1338-1344.

[61]Daniel Mowrey, Ph.D., "Ho Shou Wu: The Facts, the Frauds, the Future," *The Herbalist,* Vol. V, No. 1, 14-15, 1980.

[62]"Two for the Price of a Potato," *Alternatives,* July, 1989, 6.

[63]*Nutrition News,* Vol. XI, No. 2, 1988.

[64]*The Herbalist,* Vol. II, No. 3, 1977.

[65]*Herbal Gram,* No. 17, Summer 1988, 12.

[66]*Herbal Information Services,* 6739 West 44th Avenue, Wheat Ridge, Co., 80033, 1984.

[67]Steven Foster, "Saw Palmetto," *Health Foods Business,* April, 1992, 22-23.

[68]Betty Karmen, Ph.D., "Bee Pollen: From Principles to Practice," *Health Foods Business,* April 1991, 67.

[69]James F. Scheer, "Bee Pollen: Worth its Weight in Gold," *Health Freedom News,* October, 1990, 18-19.

[70]U. Schweinger et al., "Everyday eating behavior and menstrual function in young women," *Fertility and Sterility* 57 (1992): 771-75.

[71]"Fruit of the Womb," *Alternatives,* February, 1989.

[72]*The Doctors Book of Home Remedies,* Deborah Tkac, Ed. (Emmaus, PA: Rodale Press, 1990), 401.

[73]Bernie Siegel, "Love is a Medical Miracle," *Redbook,* December, 1986, 110-111, 181-184.

[74]Machelle M. Siebel, *Infertility: A Comprehensive Text* (East Norwalk, CT: Appleton & Lange, 1990) 31.

[75]John J. Stangel, *The New Fertility and Conception* (New York, NY: New American Library, 1988), 70.

[76]Joseph A. McFalls, Jr., *Psychopathology and Subfecundity* (New York, NY: Academic Press, 1979) 64.

[77]Joseph A. McFalls, Jr., *Psychopathology and Subfecundity* (New York, NY: Academic Press, 1979) 58.

[78]Ibid., 59.

[79]Ibid., 59.

[80]"Macho Macho Man," *East West Journal,* September 1985.

[81]Joseph A. McFalls, Jr., *Psychopathology and Subfecundity* (New York, NY: Academic Press, 1979) 93.

[82]Ibid., 65.

[83]Robert M.L. Winston, *What We Know About Infertility: Diagnosis, Treatment and Alternatives* (New York, NY: The Free Press, 1987).

[84]Cynthia Moekle, "Calm Perseverance," *American Health,* January/February, 1990), 116.

[85]Machelle M. Siebel, *Infertility: A Comprehensive Text* (East Norwalk, CT: Appleton & Lange, 1990), 33.

[86]Joseph A. McFalls, Jr., *Psychopathology and Subfecundity* (New York, NY: Academic Press, Inc., 1979) 97.

[87]Norman Cousins, "The Laughter Connection," *East West*, February, 1990, 59.

[88]Tom Ferguson, "A Psychological Journal as Self-Care: A Conversation with Ira Progoff, Ph.D.," in *Medical Self Care: Access to Health Tools*, Tom Ferguson, Ed. (New York, NY: Summit Books, 1980), 239.

Index